Dr. Sebi's Alkaline and Anti-Inflammatory Diet

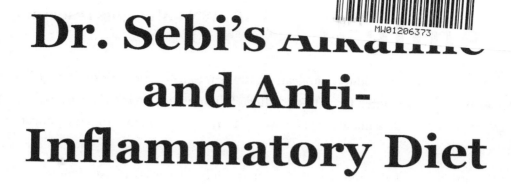

How to Naturally Reduce Inflammation and Boost Immunity for Life-Long Health | Alkaline Plant-Based Recipes, 28-Day Detox Plan & More!

SERENA BROWN

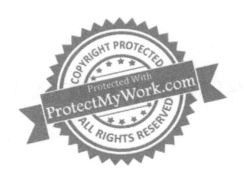

TABLE OF CONTENTS

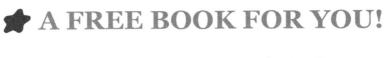 A FREE BOOK FOR YOU!
(DOWNLOAD IT) ⭐

- Are you interested in **getting rid of toxins** and nourishing your body?
- Are you curious about how Dr. Sebi used to **face disease and strengthen the immune system**?

SCAN THE QR CODE BELOW AND DISCOVER HOW TO CLEANSE YOUR WHOLE BODY IN JUST 7 DAYS!

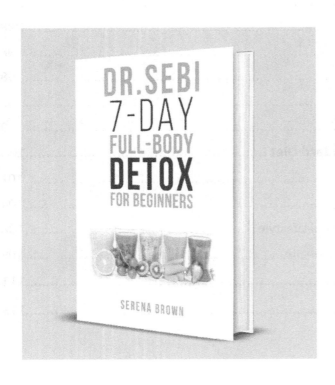

⭐ WHAT TO DO NOW ⭐

At this point, I guess you can't wait to start reading this book and learn every aspect of the true alkaline lifestyle inspired by Dr. Sebi. But first, do these two things!

STEP 1: Scan the QR Code on the previous page and learn the basics of detoxifying the body using Dr. Sebi's approved methods. After reading that, everything explained in the book will be easier to understand.

STEP 2: Let me know how excited you are about having this book in your hands!

SCAN THE QR CODE BELOW AND <u>LEAVE A QUICK REVIEW ON AMAZON</u> TO SHARE YOUR EXCITEMENT WITH THE FAMILY!

The best way to do it? **Upload a brief video** with you **talking about how you feel about it!**

SCAN ME

Is it too much for you? Not a problem at all! **A review with a couple of photos of the book would still be very nice of you!**

<u>NOTE:</u> You don't have to feel obligated, but it would be highly appreciated!

Introduction

Dr. Sebi is the inspiration for the alkaline diet. He was a natural healer from Honduras, recognized as an herbalist and an intracellular therapist. His diet is influenced by his home nation. It contains a broad range of natural alkaline foods which assist in reducing the negative effects of excessive acidity levels in the body. He created the eating plan after doing significant study and learning how acidic levels affect the body & why it's crucial to defend the body from acid levels & mucus that may lead to numerous illnesses.

Several people's lives have been enriched by his teachings, which have aided in promoting healthy living. For example, he developed an alkaline food plan that helped treat the most life-threatening disorders and helped reduce the danger of such diseases. It also assisted patients in better coping with their illnesses. As a result, the alkaline diet is effective for weight reduction and for treating ailments such as diabetes, epilepsy, arthritis, cancer, and sometimes even AIDS. Dr. Sebi spent more than 40 years investigating how alkaline foods may help people live healthier lives. He ultimately developed a nutrition plan that helps people lose weight and heal their bodies from the inside out.

We need to modify the lifestyle that Western globalization has disseminated. Hybrids, GMO meat, milk products, packaged foods, & plant foods are the primary targets. Alkaline plant foods are recommended. We need to revert to a diet that concentrates on whole, non-hybrid plant-based foods to promote the healing and balance of all organs and functions. It's the foundation of both health and medicine. We should reuse natural, vital, and non-hybrid plant elements to speed up the cure or reversal of complicated disorders. According to Dr. Sebi, Herbal therapy is vital in reviving the belief that non-hybrid plant foods have chemical elements beneficial to the body and restore health. The

African mineral balance treatment approach is based on the concept that any meal that raises the body's acidity and generates excess mucus formation is the basis of the disease.

In other words, meals high in acids and toxins infiltrate the body, triggering long-term inflammatory responses and chronic inflammation. Inflammation during sleep is a healthy, natural process that helps the body fight illness and restore physical damage. If acute inflammation is not treated, it affects healthy cells in numerous body sections, resulting in various disorders. For example, it impacts the mucosa of the protecting organs. It stimulates excessive mucus generation, compromising the health of the organs.

As a result, we must start eliminating certain things from our diet, particularly meat, dairy, and artificial hybrid foods. Although you may lose weight by adopting Dr. Sebi's diet, it is not intended to be a weight-loss plan. Western cuisine isn't designed for your meal; it's full of salt, sweet, fat, and calorie-dense fried items. A plant-based diet is advised in its stead.

Eliminate the mucous if you wish to end the sickness. Order certain "electric" foods and agree to ingest these substances to remain alive. He paid special attention to pH values and said alkaline foods were more vibrant. The alkali plus viscous idea has multiple flaws. Lastly, the immune system creates mucus to combat illness, and our acid production is necessary for cardiovascular digestion and breathing.

Dr. Sebi's life was tumultuous, and many individuals considered his ideas were harmful in some manner. However, he was audacious enough to proclaim out loud that he could discover a solution for deadly illnesses such as cancer, AIDS, and diabetes, which had eluded medical study for years. His major goal was to persuade people to live a healthy lifestyle and recognize the relevance of alkaline foods in a balanced diet. People assumed Dr. Sebi was attempting to trick them into becoming vegans, and he suffered a lot of anger as a result. But, after people saw how efficient his techniques were, he became a celebrity and one of the most well-known herbalists in the world.

Chapter 1: Dr. Sebi

Who Was Dr. Sebi?

Alfredo Bowman, commonly known as Dr. Sebi, was a self-taught herbalist born in Honduras. He went to the U.S and then was inadequately treated for diabetes, asthma, frailty, and obesity, among other chronic diseases. Finally, according to his website, an herbalist in Mexico cured him, inspiring him to make his personal herbal concoctions, which he termed Dr. Sebi's Cell Food.

Dr. Sebi's life was tumultuous, and many individuals considered his ideas were detrimental in some manner. He was audacious enough to declare publicly that he could discover a solution for deadly illnesses such as cancer, AIDS, as well as diabetes, which had eluded medical study for years. He initially claimed that his herbs might treat chronic diseases, including AIDS, sickle cell anemia, and lupus. He was jailed in 1987 for practicing medicine without a license (however, the court acquitted him). Sebi consented to avoid making claims that his medicines might heal any ailments after another litigation by the state of New York a few years later.

His major goal was to persuade people to live a healthy lifestyle and recognize the relevance of alkaline foods in a balanced diet. People assumed Dr. Sebi was attempting to trick them into becoming vegans, and he suffered a lot of criticism as a result. But, after people saw how efficient his techniques were, he became a sensation and one of the best-known herbalists in the world.

Among the many allegations leveled against Dr. Sebi, one was carried all the way to court. This claim was made in response to a 1988 commercial claiming to heal patients of fatal diseases. The Court thought they had a good case and intended to imprison him. However, a whopping 77 individuals appeared in court, claiming to have been healed after adopting Dr. Sebi's instructions and integrating his diet into their daily routines. According to the witnesses, 77 individuals declared him not responsible. They also highlighted that his diet plan was a medical marvel and undervalued.

Sebi's clientele allegedly included Michael Jackson, John Travolta, and Steven Seagal despite the controversy. He caught pneumonia while imprisoned in Honduras and starved to death in the hospital. Life went on, yet people never forgot regarding Dr. Sebi and his incredible healing abilities.

Dr. Sebi's Teachings

When toxins plus mucus build up in the body, the body becomes more vulnerable to illness. Therefore, he claimed that those suffering from various ailments and those involved in disease prevention should constantly consume an alkaline diet, keeping in mind that the body becomes free of diseases when the increasing quantity of acidic chemicals and mucus is removed.

He also claimed that bodily cleaning and detoxification is important and required technique for dealing with any ailment in the body.

Purification of the body aids in eliminating mucus collected in the liver, lungs, and many other bodily organs and the removal of excess acidic chemicals, making the body disease-free. Dr. Sebi also used herbs beneficial to the body's re-energizing and revitalization.

When human health improves, the body's organs function adequately, showing that the body is free of ailments.

Food classification by Dr. Sebi

Food was divided into six categories by Dr. Sebi:

1. Drugs

2. Food that has been genetically modified

3. Hybrid foods

4. Defunct foods

5. Living foods

6. Raw foods

He concluded that the first 4 food groups on this list should be avoided since they bring more harm than benefit to the body. For example, acids & mucus might build up in the body due to these foodstuffs. However, the remaining two kinds of foods he defined as healthy are the greatest since the nutritious value is not compromised in any manner. Foods that have been extensively cooked, hybridized, or modified, for example, have lost the needed quantity of nutrients. As a result, rather than providing health advantages, the body suffers. Raw foods, particularly vegetables, fruits, & herbs, are, on the other hand, beneficial for maintaining good health.

Dr. Sebi's Point of View

The world is growing more afflicted with debilitating diseases that directly consequence the addictive, poisonous, industrially-processed foods that indicate the Standard Diet.

The African Bio-Mineral Balance Protocol was created by Dr. Sebi to tackle the chronic health difficulties caused by contemporary diets' inadequate nutrition.

Mucus & Acidification

Dr. Sebi realized that illness is a sign of the body's deposition of mucus & acid. He was certain that just one disease is caused by consuming acidic foods. The body must take minerals from bones to reinstate alkalinity once it becomes acidic. Mucus is generated to protect cellular membranes against acidic erosion. The cell's capacity to absorb nutrients and eliminate poisonous waste products is hampered by impaired membranes and sticky mucus. Blood flow is hindered, pressure rises, oxygenation drops, and waste builds up. This creates ideal circumstances for diseases to develop because the body's natural healing processes cannot function efficiently without appropriate nourishment.

Electrification

Most foods that we assume organic have been genetically modified in labs to modify their electrical characteristics. "Cell nutrition needs to be electrical," he said, "since the body of humans is electrical." "For chemical affinity to exist, the food must be electrical."

Consequently, we resist and warn against using genetically engineered organisms (GMOs). Plants genetically modified plants lack the chemical

14

affinity that allows humans to absorb their nutrients. Real plants, created by Mother Nature, supply the body with all of the minerals and nutrients it needs to survive in an easily absorbed form.

Nourishment & Cleansing

The African Bio-Mineral Balance Program was created by Dr. Sebi to address difficulties impacting the nutrition of the African genome while also providing significant nourishment for the entire human community.

On two levels, the Balance Diet works:

- On an intracellular level, it removes toxins and mucous from the body & organs.

- Second, it replenishes the human body with the minerals required for normal electrical activity and alkalinity.

Dietary adjustments are also encouraged as part of the program to help you on your path to self-healing. Dr. Sebi recommends a plant-based diet rich in nutrient-dense vegetables, nuts, seeds, fruits, and herbs to replenish the body and preserve the alkaline balance essential for optimal health.

Eating Organic Foods: A Philosophical Approach

You should be consuming a broad range of plant-based foods. He does not push you to adopt a vegan diet, even if he feels it is sensible to solve all of your health issues. This alkaline diet's main emphasis is on eating natural and nutritious foods, which allows your body to reduce its acidic level and recover from within. Consuming the alkaline diet is based on the idea that the metabolic system would work properly again. Once the body has significant acidic content, it disrupts your metabolic system, which means that much of the food you consume is stored as fat instead of being converted into energy. While the acid levels are at their highest, it's challenging for the metabolism to function properly, creating issues with the digestive system. Suppose you really want to lead a healthier life. In that case, you must start consuming foods that help with digestion so that your physiological functions might work properly.

The first step involves improving your metabolism and converting the food you consume into energy instead of storing it as fat in the body. Your pH level begins to balance when you begin consuming nutritious meals. This process is slow, but it gradually shifts you toward an alkaline lifestyle, which is beneficial in the long term. Natural food philosophy states that you should not skip meals to lose weight but instead incorporate foods abundant in calcium and magnesium, and natural fat to alkalize the body. While you maintain a healthy regular diet, you reap many advantages that enhance your body and make you feel much better.

What are Dr. Sebi's eight diet rules?

Rule 1: Only consume the items mentioned in the nutritional guide.

Rule 2: Every day, consume 1 gallon (3.8 liters) of water.

Rule 3: Consume Dr. Sebi's pills one hour before taking your medication.

Rule 4: There are no animal products allowed.

Rule 5: No alcoholic beverages are permitted.

Rule 6: Limit wheat products as well as stick to the guide's list of "natural-growing grains."

Rule 7: If you don't want to kill your meal, don't use the microwave.

Rule 8: Stay away from canned and seedless fruits.

Chapter 2: The Alkaline Diet

The alkaline diet is designed to help adjust the pH of the fluids in the body, such as the urine and blood. Therefore, this diet is also known as the alkaline ash eating plan, alkaline acid diet, acidic ash diet, pH diet, and Dr. Sebi's alkaline diet. The diet is based on the African Bio-Mineral Balance philosophy and was created by self-taught herbalist Alfredo Darrington Bowman, known as Dr. Sebi.

He created this diet for anybody who wants to organically treat or prevent sickness while improving their general health without depending on Western medicine. As per Dr. Sebi, diseases are caused by mucus build-up in a certain body location. For instance, pneumonia is caused by the accumulation of mucus in the lungs. Still, diabetes is caused by excessive mucus in the pancreas. He claims that diseases cannot survive in an alkaline condition. They begin to manifest themselves when the body gets too acidic. Therefore, he claims to revive the body's natural alkaline condition and cleanse your sick body by rigorously adopting his diet and utilizing his patented supplements.

Dr. Sebi originally stated that this diet might treat AIDS, sickle cell anemia, leukemia, and lupus. However, following a lawsuit in 1993, he was forced to stop making such assertions.

A precise list of vegetables, fruits, cereals, hazelnuts, seeds, oils, and herbs is allowed in the diet. The Dr. Sebi program is vegan since animal products aren't allowed. According to Sebi, for the body to repair itself, you must stick to the diet for the long - term.

Finally, although many individuals say that the method has helped them recover, no scientific studies support their claims.

The Alkalinity Quest

Sebi's primary idea seems to be that alkaline foods and herbs (pH > 7) are required to manage acid in the body and that sustaining this alkaline condition protects us against disease-causing mucus build-up. Alkalinity's consecration as our long-awaited rescuer reveals a fundamental ignorance of the human body. The pH of our blood cannot be changed greatly; in fact, blood includes carbonic acid & sodium bicarbonate molecules that are particularly designed to regulate the pH between 7.35 & 7.45. Then there's disease and death. On the other hand, Sebi continued to market a broad range of herbal extracts despite that piece of high school biology.

How Does The Alkaline Diet Work?

Here's some information on acidity and alkalinity in the diet of humans, as well as some essential aspects regarding how alkaline diets might assist:

Once it comes to the overall acid content of the human diet, researchers think "there have been significant shifts from hunter-gatherer societies to the present." In comparison to diets of the past 200 years, the food supply contains far less potassium, magnesium, & chloride, and significantly more salt, thanks to the agricultural revolution & subsequent vast industrialization of the food supply.

The kidneys generally keep our electrolyte levels in check (calcium, magnesium, potassium & sodium). These electrolytes are utilized to fight acidity when subjected to highly acidic substances.

According to a study, the potassium-to-sodium proportion in most people's diets has shifted dramatically. Then, potassium seemed to dominate sodium by a factor of 10:1, but currently, the ratio is 1:3. Those who follow a "Standard American Diet" generally ingest three times as much salt as potassium! This considerably adds to our bodies' alkaline environment. Most adults and children nowadays eat high-sodium diets deficient in antioxidants, fiber, vital vitamins, and magnesium and potassium. Furthermore, processed fats, simple carbohydrates, salt, and chloride are abundant in the average Western diet.

These dietary modifications have led to a rise in "metabolic acidosis." To put it another way, many people's pH levels are no longer appropriate. Furthermore, many people have inadequate food intake and issues like potassium and magnesium deficiencies.

Health Advantages

Because alkaline meals include key elements that aid in the prevention of premature aging and the loss of organs & cellular functioning, as stated below as well, alkaline diet advantages may include assisting in the prevention of tissue and bone deterioration, which may be harmed when excessive acidity depletes us of essential minerals.

1. Bone mass & muscle mass are protected

Mineral intake is critical for the formation and preservation of bone structures. According to research, the more alkaline fruits and veggies a person consumes, the less likely they will develop sarcopenia or a loss of bone strength & muscle mass as they age. In addition, an alkaline diet may help with bone health by regulating the proportion of minerals like calcium, magnesium, and phosphate, which are necessary for forming bones and preserving lean muscle mass.

The diet might even aid in the synthesis of growth hormones and the consumption of vitamin D, which preserves bones while also reducing the risk of many other chronic illnesses.

2. Reduces Hypertension & Stroke Risk

Reduced inflammation and increased growth hormone production are two of the anti-aging benefits of an alkaline diet. This has been demonstrated to boost cardiovascular health and protect against excessive cholesterol, high blood pressure, kidney problems, stroke, and sometimes even memory loss.

3. Reduces Inflammation and Chronic Pain

According to research, an alkaline diet has been linked to lower levels of chronic pain. Backaches, headaches, muscular spasms, menstruation symptoms, inflammation, and joint pain have all been linked to persistent acidosis.

According to research, people with chronic back pain who were administered an alkaline tablet daily for four weeks reported substantial reductions in pain as evaluated by the "Arhus low back pain assessment scale," according to research.

4. Helps to prevent Magnesium Deficiency by increasing vitamin absorption

Magnesium is necessary for the proper functioning of thousands of enzyme systems and biological functions. Unfortunately, many individuals are magnesium deficient, resulting in heart problems, muscular pains, migraines, sleep problems, and anxiety. Magnesium is also needed to stimulate vitamin D and avoid vitamin D insufficiency, critical for general immunological and endocrine health.

5. Assists in the strengthening of immune function and the prevention of cancer

If cells have little or no minerals, they need to dump waste effectively or adequately oxygenate the whole body's struggles. Mineral loss impairs vitamin absorption, while toxins and infections build up in the body, weakening the immune system. An alkaline change in pH owing to an adjustment in electric charges and the discharge of primary elements of proteins is thought to be linked to cancer prevention. Alkalinity has been demonstrated to be more advantageous for certain chemotherapeutic medicines that need a higher pH to act properly and reduce inflammation and the risk of conditions like cancer.

6. It may assist you in maintaining a healthy weight

Although the diet isn't primarily for weight reduction, sticking to an alkaline diet dietary pattern for weight loss will assist you in avoiding becoming obese. Due to the diet's tendency to lower leptin levels and inflammation, limiting acid-forming meals and consuming greater alkaline-forming foods might make it simpler to lose weight. This has an impact on your appetite as well as your fat-burning ability.

Because alkaline-forming foods are anti-inflammatory, following an alkaline diet allows your body to attain normal leptin levels and feel full with eating the right calorie count.

How to Follow It?

1. Purchase organic alkaline foods wherever feasible.

One crucial factor in adopting an alkaline diet, according to experts, is to learn about the sort of soil your food was produced in since fruits and vegetables cultivated in organic, mineral-dense soil are more alkalizing. However, according to research, the kind of soil in which plants are cultivated greatly impacts their vitamin & mineral content; therefore, not all "alkaline foods" are made equal.

For the best adequate amount of vital nutrients in plants, the pH of the soil should be between 6 and 7. Acidic soils with a pH below 6 may have lower calcium and magnesium levels. In contrast, soils with a pH of more than 7 may contain chemically inaccessible iron, manganese, copper, and zinc. In addition, the healthiest soil is well-rotated, organically supported, and vulnerable to wildlife/grazing cattle.

2. Consume alkaline water.

The pH of alkaline water ranges from 9 to 11. Therefore, it's perfectly safe to consume distilled water. Although reverse osmosis filtered water is somewhat acidic, it is still preferable to tap water or purified bottled water. Alkalinity may also be increased by adding lime to drinking water.

3. Measure your pH level (optional)

You may test your pH level by buying strips at the local health food shop or pharmacy if you're wondering about the pH level before adopting the instructions below. Saliva or urine may be used to determine your pH.

The finest benefits will come from your second urination of the morning. The colors on the test strip are compared to a chart included with the test strip kit. 1 hour before a meal and 2 hours after a meal is the optimum times to test your pH throughout the day. If you're testing your saliva, aim for a reading of 6.8 to 7.2.

Is It Safe To Follow An Alkaline Diet?

The alkaline diet is essentially a reinforcement of excellent, ancient healthy habits. The diet encourages people to consume more vegetables, fruits, and water while avoiding sweets, alcohol, meat, especially processed meals. All of these factors would help you improve your general health, lose weight, and even reduce your cancer risk — but not for the purposes that diet proponents claim.

This diet may also aid in the reduction of inflammation. Although inflammation is a normal reaction to injury and illness, too much inflammation, usually known as chronic inflammation, may damage DNA & lead to cancer. As a result, consuming anti-inflammatory foods may help lower your cancer risk.

Foods to Avoid

The pH of specific foods is used to regulate the diet. Some variants are less rigorous, allowing grains despite their moderately acidic pH for health advantages. However, if you're on an alkaline diet, you would like to stick to the list of foods below, limiting acidic meals, limiting or eliminating neutral foods, and concentrating on alkaline foods.

Foods to Stay Away From

- Meat products

- Poultry

- Fish

- Milk

- Cheese

- Yogurt

- Ice-cream

- Eggs (especially the yolk of the egg)

- Grain products (rice (brown & white), rolled oats, pasta, cornflakes, rye & whole-wheat bread)

- Alcohol

- Soda

- Lentils

- Walnuts plus peanuts

- Other cooked, packaged foods

Limiting Neutral Foods

- Natural fats including oil (olive), cream, butter

- Starches

- Sugars

- Foods to Consume That Are Alkaline

- Fruit

- Fruit juices that haven't been sweetened

- Raisins

- Currants, black

- Veggies (especially kale)

- Potatoes

- Wine

- Soda water with minerals

- Soy-based foods

- Legumes

- Seeds

- Nuts

Is This What Our Forefathers ate?

The paleo diet, which aims to emulate our gatherer ancestors' nutritional patterns, has a lot of similarities with the alkaline diet's focus on fruits and vegetables over manufactured meals. However, the evidence does not necessarily support the notion that our forefathers ate alkaline diets. According to an earlier study, almost half of the 229 ancient diets studied constituted acid-producing, whereas the other half constituted alkaline-forming.

Another research revealed that the disparity might be due to location. The researchers discovered that the further individuals lived from the equator, the greater acidic the diets were.

Principles of an Alkaline Diet

Most people find it challenging to eat healthily. However, with all of the food options available, it's critical to keep concentrated on what matters most — your health! "The Alkaline Way" is based on seven principles. Employ these principles to build and experience an Alkaline Diet that is delicious and healthful.

1. Consume a diverse range of fresh, high-quality whole foods.

The first principle in perusing the Alkaline Way is to consume mostly whole foods. This is the foundation of the Alkaline Diet. Fresh fruit and veggies, gently roasted nuts and seeds, slightly cooked vegetables, grain & bean sprouts, cultured foods, freshly squeezed juices, as well as vegetable juices must all be high on your list of "life-ly" foods. These foods are high inactive enzymes, which help indigestion.

Eat a broad range of whole foods to get the most health benefits. When digestion is poor, agitated, or weakened, consuming the same foods repeatedly restricts digestive and nutritional diversity and raises the risk of being allergic to those foods. Instead, diversify your diet selections to include items that are simple to digest, absorb, and remove. Experiment with different flavors—and you'll frequently get a health benefit in the process.

2. Consume 60-80% alkaline-forming foods.

The second principle is to eat mostly alkaline foods. If you are in excellent health, it is suggested that you consume at least 60percent alkaline-forming foods. Experts recommend an 80 percent alkalinizing diet to assist in soothing the immune system and improving digestion if the immune system is impaired or responding to anything or if the health requires to be preserved in any manner.

3. Consume foods that are good for your immune system.

Avoiding foods that cause your immune system to respond is the 3rd Alkaline Method principle for eating healthy. When overweight persons replace reactive foods with nonreactive foods and follow the Alkaline Way, they lose weight easily (even if they consume more calories), and their metabolism improves. On the other hand, most underweight persons achieve a healthy weight due to a health-promoting diet that boosts protein synthesis and repair.

4. Consume 60-70% plant-based, complex carbohydrates; 15-20% protein; and 15-20% healthy fat.

The fourth Alkaline Method principle promotes a balanced ratio of complex carbs, proteins, and fats. Ratios to Consider:

- Whole food (plant-based) complex carbs provide 60–70% calories.

- Protein accounts for 15–20 percent of total calories.

- Healthy fats account for 15–20 percent of calories (including most of the omega-3 fats)

Complex Carbohydrates from Whole Foods (Plant-Based)

Your Alkaline Way meal plan should be high in complex carbs from veggies, whole grains, plus legumes (beans, peas, & lentils). Also, spices, seasonings, and herbs, except the healthcare professional advise differently. 60-70 percent of your daily calories should come from these sources.

Beneficial fats:

Fat should account for 15-20% of the caloric intake. So make sure to eat enough omega-3 healthy fats, which help your body produce energy, protein, as well as rebuild tissue. Fresh nuts and seeds and cold-pressed natural oils are food-based resources of beneficial omega-3 essential fats.

Combining foods to make complete proteins:

Plant proteins, unlike animal proteins, lack some necessary amino acids. Therefore, you can get a complete protein by combining meals depending on the amino acid content. Brown rice and roasted beans, for example, are insufficient proteins when consumed alone because they lack a key amino acid; yet, while eaten simultaneously, they support each other and constitute a full protein intake.

The body treats "trans" fatty acids as if they had been naturally saturated fats such as butter and coconut oil, yet these fats are more dangerous. Tran's fats penetrate the placenta, are preserved in fetal tissue and may affect cell membrane functioning in the long run. However, "trans" fats may be found in fried meals like French fries, as well as many processed foods, including anything from name-brand oils to bakery products and confectionery.

Use unsaturated, non-hydrogenated "expeller-pressed" oils such as olive, grape seed, coconut, peanut, and exotic oils like avocado.

Hydrogenated oils have increased cholesterol levels and interference with liver enzymes. In addition, these synthetic oils are also known to harm immunological function and encourage the growth of some kinds of malignancies.

5. Consume foods and beverages that are probiotic and fermented (cultured).

The Alkaline Way's fifth principle is to establish a habit of eating and drinking a wide variety of probiotics (cultured/fermented) foods and beverages. The word probiotic refers to a bacterium that aids in the growth of living organisms. A normal gastrointestinal tract is a home to a diverse range of beneficial (probiotic) bacteria that help maintain the balance of the body and immune systems. Poor nutrition, stress, illnesses, and medications may reduce good bacteria, allowing infections to flourish. Probiotics are used to populate the stomach with good microorganisms.

Probiotics should be consumed in food or drink since this gives the maximum amounts and diversity of probiotics.

6. Drink plenty of water and consume plenty of fiber.

The 6th Alkaline Way principle is to drink enough water and eat plenty of fiber. Ordinary people drink far too little water and eat far too little fiber. Traditional civilizations ingest 40-100 grams of dietary fiber per day from real, active foods to avoid developing Western degenerative illnesses. Fiber's "roughage" makes the stool thick and mushy, which focuses on maintaining a reduced transit time—the frequency between eating and eliminating waste. Adequate fiber supports waste elimination daily simply and comfortably. It's less probable that poisonous waste would be recycled back into circulation if you keep the body clean and clear.

A good transit time is between 12 and 18 hours. This minimizes the chances of harmful germs and yeast taking over the body.

Water and its importance:

Drinking enough water is essential for good health, particularly if you eat a high-fiber diet. Water aids fiber in effectively passing wastes thru the body, and water is required for the proper functioning of every system in the body. Experts suggest drinking a minimum of one 8-ounce glass of filtered water eight times a day while implementing The Alkaline Way plan.

7. Consume more nutritious food combinations.

The Alkaline Way's last principle is effective food mixing, a crucial element of the Alkaline Way. The way we mix meals at mealtime may significantly influence digestion and, as a result, general health.

The skill of healthy meal combining is an essential part of balanced nutrition since it reduces digestive system wear and strain. If you're prone to stomach issues, pay special attention to how you combine foods (acid reflux, cramping, leaky gut syndrome, indigestion, irritable bowel syndrome, diverticulosis, as well as other digestive issues).

The Importance of a Balanced PH

The lungs and kidneys are mostly responsible for keeping the body's pH in check, and it's a fine line to tread. The pH of the blood varies from 7.2 to 7.45. The kidneys also aid in the pH balance of urine. For example, a urine pH of 4 indicates that it is very acidic. In contrast, a pH of 7 indicates that it is neutral, and a pH of 9 indicates strongly alkaline.

ause excessive acid may be ejected via the urine to rectify the body's pH levels.

If the body's pH fluctuates, it's a sign of a major health problem. For example, urine with a high pH may suggest a UTI or kidney stones. In contrast, urine with a low pH may indicate diarrhea, hunger, or diabetic ketoacidosis.

What is "pH Level," and What Does It Mean?

The potency of hydrogen is referred to as pH. It's a measurement of the acidity and alkalinity of the fluids and tissues in our bodies. It's assessed from 0 – 14 on a scale of 1 to 14. The lower the pH of a solution, the more acidic it is. The higher the value, the more alkaline the body is. A pH of approximately 7 is considered neutral; however, since the normal human body pH is around 7.4, we perceive a little alkaline pH to be the best.

The stomach is the most acidic part of the body, with varying pH values. Thus, even little changes in the pH of many organisms may create serious difficulties. For example, the ocean's pH has reduced from 8.2 to 8.1 due to environmental problems such as increased CO_2 deposition, and numerous ocean living organisms have suffered considerably as a result.

The pH level is really important for plant growth. Thus it has a huge effect on the mineral composition of the meals we consume. Nutrients in the ocean, soil, and human body act as buffers to keep pH levels in check; therefore, as acidity rises, minerals decline.

Acidity

What precisely is acidity?

The pH scale determines whether a substance is acidic, basic, or neutral.

- A pH level of 0 implies a strong acidity level.

- A pH level of 7 is considered neutral.

- A pH level of 14 seems to be the most basic/alkaline.

A tenfold imbalance in acidity and alkalinity of content is represented by the distance among two points upon the pH scale. The acidity of a pH level of 6 is 10 times that of a pH of 7, & so on. Acidity, as well as alkalinity, are measured using the pH scale. It determines if a solution contains both positively & negatively charged hydrogen ions. The more the hydrogen ions, the more acidic the solution.

Foods with a pH of 4.6 or below are considered acidic. This is because foods high in acid are far less to promote rapid microorganism development. Therefore they may take longer to break down.

The Human Body and Acidity

The pH of the body is around 7.40. This level is ideal for keeping the body's biochemical functions running smoothly. Blood oxygenation is among the most critical activities it regulates.

Despite the lack of compelling evidence that this helps maintain normal pH levels, many people choose to avoid meals that increase acidity in the stomach. Their major objective is to maintain their PRAL (potential renal acid load) under control. When you consume particular meals, your body creates a certain amount of acid, measured by the PRAL.

Excessive body acidity is regarded to become the first step in premature aging, vision and memory problems, wrinkling, age spots, hormone system failure, and a slew of other age-related issues. In addition, body acidity is linked to practically most diseases.

We get more acidic as we become older. Most elderly people's bodies are very acidic, with hazardous wastes accumulating in the bloodstream, tissues, and lymphatic system. Acidic wastes arise from a variety of places. Therefore, you could substantially slow down the aging process if you kept your skin, muscles, organs, as well as glands alkaline as they were when you were an infant.

The following are the first indications of acidity in bodily tissues:

- Feeling tired, weak, and short on energy

- Irritability, anxiety, panic attacks, and despair

- Having skin conditions such as eczema, psoriasis, acne, and hives

- Experiencing widespread aches and pains

- Diarrhea, constipation, or stomach pain

- Experiencing cramps before or during your period

- Feelings of heartburn

- Sleep deprivation

- Having an increased dental decay

- Feeling nauseous

- Experiencing libido loss

Long-term bodily acidity manifests itself in a variety of ways, including:

- Osteoporosis

- Immune system dysfunction

- Consistent digestive issues

- Arthritis, ligament and joint disorders

- Gout, kidney stones, and kidney disorders

- Problems with the heart and circulation

- Infections caused by fungi and bacteria

- Cancers

Avoid acidic foods

These items are acid-forming, and their consumption should be avoided as part of a healthy diet:

- Convenience foods

- Alcohol

- Milk

- Caffeinated beverages

- Cereals that have been processed

- Pizza

- Sweeteners made from artificial sources

- Peanuts

- Cheese

- Pasta

- Rice

- Bread

- Products made from wheat

- Butter

- Cold cuts

- Vegetable oils that have been refined

- French fries

- Hot chocolate

- Red meat
- Beverages for sports
- Sugar (table)

- Corn syrup
- Pancakes
- Fried Foods

What is Acidosis?

Acidosis is a condition in which the body's acid levels are extraordinarily high. For optimum health, the body must achieve a balance of acidity. Too much acidity or alkalinity in the body may lead to major health concerns. When the body's acid levels are too high, it tries to adjust by removing the acid. Excessive acid in the body is normally excreted via the lungs and kidneys. Acidosis may produce major consequences if it puts excessive strain on these organs. Acidosis may be caused by various medical disorders, prescription medicines, and dietary variables. Although some forms of acidosis may be reversed, acute acidosis can be deadly if not treated.

Excessive acidity compromises the health of all physiological systems. To buffer (neutralize) the acid & safely eliminate it from the body, the body borrows minerals such as calcium, salt, potassium, and magnesium from essential organs, bones, and teeth. As a consequence of the excessive acidity, the body might suffer severe and long-term corrosion. This condition can go unnoticed for years. In addition, acidosis may cause catastrophic difficulties in key organs, including the liver, heart, and kidneys.

It causes obesity and diabetes.

An acidic pH may lead to weight issues, including diabetes and obesity. On the other hand, insulin Sensitivity is a syndrome that occurs when our bodies get excessively acidic. This causes an overabundance of insulin to be generated. Consequently, the body is bombarded with far too much insulin that each calorie is dutifully converted to fat.

An acid pH caused by an unbalanced diet is extremely likely to cause a state that triggers the planned genetic response to hunger and famine. Following that, the body will be forced to horde and store every calorie ingested as fat. Some believe that an acid pH triggers a strong genetic reaction to an imminent famine, directly interpreted by the all-important and extremely sensitive Insulin-Glucagon Axis. When this occurs, the body produces more insulin than normal, which causes the body to manufacture and retain extra fat.

A healthy, slightly alkaline pH, on either hand, will result in typical fat-burning metabolic activity, with no need for the body to manufacture additional insulin or lipids. As a result, fat may be burnt and removed naturally. A balanced pH diet is also less likely to result in yo-yo effects or weight gain after a diet. We should aim for a little alkaline pH to enable fats to be used naturally for energy rather than being hoarded and saved due to a faulty biochemical belief in a coming famine. Acidosis also damages the insulin-producing beta cells in the pancreas. The beta cells are extremely pH sensitive and cannot thrive in an acidic environment. Beta cells will lose sync with one another if this happens. Their cellular connection will be disrupted, and the body's immune system will begin to overreact. The cells' stress levels will rise, making it more difficult to function properly and live.

It hastens free radical damage as well as early aging.

Acidosis triggers lipid breakdown and harmful oxidative cascades, speeding up free radical damage to cell walls & intracellular membrane structures. Most healthy cells are killed as a result of this process.

Premature aging and enhanced oxidative pathways of cell wall degradation begin with acidosis. Wrinkling, dark circles, failed hormonal systems, interference with vision, memory, and other age-related issues are all signs of acidosis. Unwanted wastes that are not effectively expelled from the body poison the cells.

It causes lipid & fatty acid metabolism to be disrupted.

Acidosis impairs lipid & fatty acid metabolism, which is important for brain and nerve function. This disturbance results in neurological issues such as MS and MD and hormonal imbalances in the endocrine system.

In addition, an acidic environment induces LDL-cholesterol to be built down at a faster rate in the heart, lining and clogging the vascular network improperly. In other words, an acid pH causes electrostatic potential, which damages artery walls and triggers a PDGF-dependent immunological response, resulting in cholesterol oxidation and heavy metal plaque development.

It erodes the tissues of the arteries, veins, and heart.

Acidosis diminishes and eats away at the cell wall membranes of the heart, arteries, and veins, much as acid eats away at the marble. Our cardiac structures and interconnected tissues are weakened due to this erosion process.

The chemical environment of all biological tissues affects them. The cardiac muscle cells are no exception. Blood plasma pH affects the whole cardiovascular system, which functions as one vast functional "system of tubular muscles" to transport blood and nutrients to every living tissue in the body. The heart's pumping forces blood thru the arteries, veins, and capillary beds, assisting in regulating blood pressure and blood flow.

An acid pH disrupts free ionic balances in circulation, resulting in an increase in populations of positively charged particles, w

hich interferes with heart and artery muscle excitability (contraction and relaxation).

Changes in blood pH are currently considered to cause the following:

- Arteriosclerosis development (tightening of the arteries)

- Aneurysm (widening as well as ballooning of artery walls)

- Arrhythmias (irregular heart beating including tachycardia)

- Myocardial infarction (cardiovascular attacks)

- Strokes (a heart accident).

- The anatomical deterioration of the cardio-vascularity ultimately causes blood pressure anomalies, exacerbating the issues mentioned above.

It affects the metabolism and reserve of energy.

Effective cellular and overall metabolism are hampered when your body's pH is too acidic. Acidosis disrupts cellular connections and functioning by causing chemical ionic disruptions. Acidosis lowers plasma protein plus calcium-binding, lowering the efficiency of such intracellular signal. It also causes a condition characterized by the admission of calcium cations via positive calcium channels. As a result, cardiovascular contractibility, or the heart's capacity to pump effectively and rhythmically, is reduced.

The "Sodium-Potassium pump" regulates intracellular protein activity and drives positive calcium plus hydrogen from the cells (Na-K pump). This pump creates a powerful inducement for sodium to be transported into cells. It also manages the amount of sodium & potassium in the body's reserves, and it consumes up to 25% of our daily calorie intake.

Positive calcium swaps plus sodium and is pushed out of cells. In contrast, the electrolytic cell for positive calcium promotes both positive hydrogen & positive calcium entrance into cells since cells contain less calcium & positive hydrogen than extracellular fluids. Therefore, the quantity of positive sodium in extracellular fluids is ten times higher.

Because less + sodium is accessible in acidic liquids, the digestion and induction of nutritious elements entering the cells are slow. This increases the amount of positive hydrogen plus calcium in the plasma, enabling LDL-Cholesterol to attach electrostatically. Due to the disruption of free positive calcium communities and channels, calcium may be excessively siphoned from bone masses. Osteoporosis is the result of this. In a word, an acidic pH depletes our energy stores and prevents us from using them.

It reduces the rate at which oxygen is delivered to the cell.

Acidosis lowers the amount of oxygen in the blood. Because all living tissues, particularly the heart and brain, need oxygen to thrive, a shortage will result in death. In addition, the quantity of oxygen given to the cells is reduced when the pH is acidic. As a result, they will perish at some point.

Acidosis is linked to a variety of diseases

It's vital to remember that the body's biochemistry is simply one of several tools that a physician may use to better comprehend the whole body. A pH result is neither a diagnostic tool nor a clinical diagnosis of any problem on its own. What happens if the body becomes excessively acidic? When you have an acidic balance, you'll be able to:

- Reduce the capacity of the body to retain minerals as well as other substances

- Reduce the amount of energy produced by the cells.

- Reduce the capacity of the body to fix the damaged cells

- Reduce the ability of the body to cleanse heavy metals

- Enable the tumor cells to proliferate.

- Increase your body's susceptibility to tiredness and diseases.

Anxiousness, diarrhea, dilated pupils, gregarious behavior, exhaustion in the morning, headaches, impulsivity, hypersexuality, sleeplessness, anxiety, racing heart, restless legs, breathlessness, sturdy appetite, hypertension, warm dry feet and hands are some of the symptoms that people with high acidity levels experience.

The body turns acidic almost all of the time due to a high-acid diet, mental stress, toxic overload, immunological responses, or any other activity that precludes the cells of oxygen & other nutrients. The body will attempt to counteract the acidic pH by consuming alkaline minerals like calcium. Unfortunately, calcium is lost from the bones, resulting in osteoporosis. Rheumatoid arthritis, diabetes, lupus, TB, osteoporosis, hypertension, and most tumors may be caused by acidosis, defined as a prolonged time in an acid pH condition.

An acidic pH, as well as oxygen deprivation, are two major causes of cancer. Cancer thrives and survives in an acidic, low-oxygen condition, as we all know. According to research, the acidity level of terminal cancer patients is 1,000 times higher than that of healthy persons. The pH level of the significant number of terminal patients is very acidic.

What is the reason behind this?

The reason is obvious. Lactic acid is formed when glucose is fermented without the presence of oxygen. The cell's pH drops to 7.0 as a result of this. The pH level drops to 6.5 in more advanced cancer situations. The level may even drop to 6.0, 5.7, or even lower occasionally. The simple reality is that human bodies cannot fight infections if our pH levels are out of whack.

The Long-Term Consequences of Living in an Acidic Medium

Structural System

While serum & soft tissue calcium levels drop, calcium held in bones is discharged, binding and neutralizing excessive acid in the tissues. Muscle cramps may result from the first calcium deficiency in the muscle. As more calcium is drawn from the bones to neutralize acid, the calcium deposits in the bones are depleted, resulting in osteoporosis, weaker and collapsed vertebrae, &, often, terrible posture and back discomfort. In addition, the calcium that is mobilized from the bones is accumulated in the joints as calcium-acid salts, causing degenerative arthritis.

Nervous System

When brain cells get overly acidic, they lose their capability to work properly. Consequently, the brain is unable to create the necessary chemicals (neurotransmitters) to interact with neighboring brain cells. As a result, sleeplessness, anxiety, melancholy, neuroses, psychotic disorders, and memory loss are possible outcomes. In addition, because the brain is meant to interact with every cell in the human body (heart cells, intestine cells, muscular cells, epithelial cells, etc.) via the spinal cord as well as other nerves, if the neurological system is not operating effectively due to acidic imbalance, every bodily system might fail.

Circulatory System

Bacteria, fungi, and/or viruses may adhere themselves to the interior wall of arteries when the pH is too high. This subsequently recruits white blood cells, coagulation proteins, clotting cells, and other clotting factors to the region. This may result in plaque formation in the artery, narrowing it and reducing the blood flow, oxygen, and nutrients into the tissues served by that artery. A heart attack occurs when the coronary artery is obstructed.

Calcium, which was recruited from the bone to neutralize the acid, may accumulate in the arterial plaque if there is a surplus of acidity, transforming the plaque from floppy to stiff. As a result, the plaque stiffens the arteries, resulting in a rise in blood pressure.

Digestive System

The cells that make up the stomach & small intestine and the cells of the pancreas involved in creating and discharging digestive enzymes do not function properly when the pH is excessively acidic. Indigestion, heartburn, bloating, and stomach cramps are all symptoms. If the body does not absorb enough nutrients from the diet, malnutrition may occur throughout the body. In addition, foods that have not been digested might develop in the intestines, producing toxicity.

Intestinal System

Increased acidity induces colon cells to malfunction, resulting in diarrhea, irritable bowel syndrome, constipation, and diverticulitis. In addition, colitis, inflammatory bowel disorder (particularly Crohn's disease), and hemorrhoids may all be caused by a disrupted acid level in the colon, which allows unfavorable microorganisms to flourish and thrive.

Immune System

Antibodies & cytokines (chemical messengers that govern other immune cells) are not produced by immune cells that are overly acidic, and phagocytosis is impeded (the capability to ingest and spoilage microorganisms). Consequently, the person is vulnerable to a viral, bacterium, fungal infections, and cancer.

Respiratory System

Oxygen adhesion to hemoglobin occurs across a very limited pH range in the lungs. Therefore, microbes in the airways may grow much more readily if the pH is excessively acidic, invading human cells and causing bronchitis, pneumonia, sinusitis, and other infections, as well as cough, bronchial spasms (asthma), and greater sensitivity to allergens (hay fever).

Urinary System

The urinary system aids in the removal of harmful waste from the body. Due to their narrower urethra, which links the urine bladder to the outside of the body, women contain bacteria and/or fungus in their bladders. If the urine pH isn't in the correct proportions, these bacteria might multiply quickly. In addition, calcium, which is recruited from the bone to moderate the acid, may create calcium crystals and stones in the kidney's collecting system when the situation is too acidic.

Glandular System

Enzymatic activity is used by all endocrine glands to create hormones. The epithelial cells cannot create and release enough hormones to meet the body's demands if the pH is excessively acidic. Changes in mood, blood sugar imbalances, exhaustion, reproductive problems, and other issues emerge due to this.

Loss of weight

The metabolic enzymes within the cells do not perform correctly when the pH is excessively acidic, preventing the effective breakdown of fats and other nutrients.

Acid indigestion is spurred by the foods we eat. Acid-rich foods reduce the pH of your blood. Unfortunately, it also causes health issues such as stone development, decreased bone strength, and even boosts cancer risk. As a result, keep an eye on your food to keep yourself protected from all of these problems. Human blood pH levels should be between 7.35 and 7.45. As a result, any foodstuff below this amount causes acid reflux. So, here are the top ten foods to avoid if you want to reduce your acidity.

1. hydrogenated vegetable oils

Hydrogenated oils are much more of a research project than food. The addition of a hydrogen molecule into monounsaturated and polyunsaturated oils necessitates a slew of compounds, heavy metals, heat, and other procedures that turn the oil incomprehensible and harmful to your cells. Vegetable oils (hydrogenated) do not rot on the shelf. The premise that they do not split naturally implies that your body will have difficulty digesting them. Don't be fooled: these meals aren't good for your heart. They must be avoided at all costs.

Oils such as coconut oil, cacao butter, olive oil (extra virgin from Greece and Italy, to ensure it hasn't been tampered with), or even pastured organic butter are beneficial for your body since they are identifiable as food.

2. Vegetable oils that have been processed

Corn, canola, and 'vegetable oils are mono & polyunsaturated fats with compounds that do not have a hydrogen molecule connected to them. This allows them to easily react with several other environmental elements, such as free radicals, light, warmth, and air. Because these oils are so easily broken down, they are almost rotten by reaching the shelves. Separating them from plants than putting them into bottles is practically difficult without inflicting damage. These oils have been artificially deodorized and processed to make them seem and smell fresh, but they are still rancid.

Naturally saturated oils such as coconut & cacao butter are good substitutes, and so are complete food sources such nuts, seeds, pecan and seed butter, avocado, and olives.

3. Standard dairy products

Traditional dairy cows are chemically fertilized for years to induce them to make milk - they are mammals, just like humans, and only produce milk once they have offspring to feed. Then, hormones, antibiotics, and other treatments are pumped into them to keep their milk production up and help them battle diseases and illnesses that they are susceptible to due to their disorders.

Because of the procedure to be rendered 'safe' for ingestion, traditional dairy is also exceedingly acidic for the body. Since your body must maintain an alkaline pH, the acidic composition of milk robs calcium and other alkaline elements from your body. When you eat acidic meals, your body uses alkaline reserves in the teeth and bones to counteract the acid, resulting in a net calcium loss. Overall, milk does not benefit the body in its present condition.

Alternatives: Choose plant-based milk such as hempseed and coconut.

4. Flour (White)

Even though it has been fortified, white flour remains nutritionally deficient. This is because the germ and bran are removed from white flour during the manufacturing process, leaving just the endosperm. In addition, the bran contains nutrient-rich oils, whereas the germ contains most vitamins and minerals. When these two items are removed from the equation, you're left with only starch.

This starch is subsequently bleached, which decreases its nutritious value even further. Finally, you have a material in your body that transforms into paper Mache, which is very acidic and devoid of nourishment. Synthetic vitamins placed back into enhanced flour might not be as well utilized by your body as organic minerals and vitamins that would've been present in the plant if it had not been treated at all.

Whole grains may be used as a substitute! Whole wheat, spelled, rye, and oat is all good choices. You might also want to try sprouted grain goods and gluten-free options – just make sure your gluten-free options aren't also completely processed & comprised of refined grains.

5. Processed foods labeled as "low fat."

When you read the phrases 'low fat' or 'fat-free' on prepared or packaged goods (this doesn't include organically low-fat foods, including fruits and vegetables), you can expect that the items have gone through numerous steps of processing and include a myriad of chemicals, preservatives, and stabilizers. Your body will not recognize these meals as nourishment, and they will not help you shrink down your waistline. What they'll do is make your body struggle overtime to break down the compounds and look for any remaining nourishment in the food. These goods are just unworthy of your body after the day.

Substitutes: Whole foods are best. Begin consuming more naturally reduced-fat foods, including whole fruits and vegetables, if you want to cut down on your fat consumption. Alternatively, consume naturally occurring fats such as nuts, seeds, avocado, and coconut, which your body will recognize and utilize to build a healthy body.

6. Aspartame

Aspartame has been identified as a neurotoxin. This implies that when you eat it, it essentially poisons your brain. It becomes more dangerous as it degrades in the presence of heat, and most aspartame-containing products have been heated via cooking or improper storage. It may be found in various foods, particularly those branded as "sugar-free." In addition, Aspartame may build up in the body over time and cause harm. The long & short of it is that you should never consume aspartame.

Natural sweeteners may be used as a substitute. Fruits, maple syrup, dates, and coconut sugar are all good options for naturally sweetened dishes.

7. Deli Meats/Hot Dogs (processed)

Meat that has been processed is not even actually meat. These are the meat in the notion that they have meat as a component, but they also contain many non-meat ingredients. The salt content in the deli and other processed meat items is quite high, which is bad for your heart. They're also loaded with toxins that are harmful to your health. Nitrates are one of the most bizarre substances found in deli slices, and they are well-known carcinogens.

8. Soda

It's largely made up of lab-created chemicals and flavored with excessive fructose corn syrup, which is known to be an empty calorie, meaning it delivers calories but no nourishment. The sugar concentration in soda, along with the absence of fiber that would typically limit the discharge of sugars in your system, will result in a large blood sugar surge. This puts a lot of strain on the liver & pancreas to get those sugars from the circulation into your cells.

Because soda is highly acidic, the body will have to draw from the alkaline mineral reserves in the bones and teeth to maintain the mild alkaline PH of the blood. And sugar-free drinks are no better: the artificial sugars in calorie-free sodas probably trigger your brain to crave sweets, causing you to consume more throughout the day than you might if you simply consumed a regular soda with regular sugar.

If you're looking for something effervescent, try kombucha, a traditional fermented tea drink. Tea, fresh juices, plus water may also assist your body stay hydrated.

9. Foods that are deep-fried

The oil that has been heated to frying temperatures is basically rancid. This is because the intense temperature denatures them and changes their chemical structure. When you mix this with the protein clumping and nutrient denaturing that occurs during the frying process, you end up with a food-like product that actually depletes your body of nutrients rather than delivering them. Therefore, fried foods must never, ever be eaten. In addition, Trans Fatty Acids are found in fried meals, and we already know that these are the fats that are the most harmful to your health. These fats are oxidized fats that induce cell damage and are associated with heart disease.

10. Genetically altered corn

You should be aware of three things: 1) Corn is grain rather than a vegetable. 2) Because humans lack the digestive enzymes required to thoroughly break down corn, it usually passes via your digestive system undamaged. 3) Pesticides have been transformed on a molecular level in GMO corn, which indicates the chemicals are not just on the ground but also part of the corn's genetic makeup.

All of this is really harmful to your health. When you consider that GMO corn is included in almost all processed goods, you may be consuming a diet mostly made up of GMO corn products. The majority of fast food buns, for example, are made out of 70-80% corn! There isn't even wheat.

Substitute: When choosing a side dish, use unprocessed bread/grain items and organic vegetables.

Other important foods to avoid includes:

- Excessive legumes

- Garlic

- Excessive nuts

- Alcohol

Approved List of Alkaline Foods by Dr. Sebi

Dr. Sebi was a fitness & wellbeing expert who developed a vegan diet centered on alkaline rather than hybrid foods. Dr. Sebi, a Honduran man from unfortunate conditions, made significant progress in the realm of natural health and wellbeing by developing his specialized diet, which contains seeded fruits (excluding seedless fruits), wild rice, syrup of agave, extra virgin olive oil, coconut oil, and other ingredients. Dr. Sebi believed in six basic food groups: living, raw, deceased, hybrid, genetically engineered, and drugs.

His diet virtually eliminated all food categories except live and raw, urging dieters to follow a vegetarian diet as precisely as possible. Foods like organically produced fruits and veggies, and whole grains fall under this category. Dr. Sebi felt that raw and living meals were "electric" and helped the body fight acidic waste. Dr. Sebi created a list of foods he felt ideal for his diet, which he dubbed the Dr. Sebi Electric Food Guide. Dr. Sebi's product line continues to expand and adapt even after death.

If you eat out frequently, adhering to the Dr. Sebi Diet & Dr. Sebi Food List might be tough. As a consequence, you should get used to cooking a large number of vegan diet foods at home (using wild rice, extra virgin olive oil, syrup of agave, etc.).

Vegetables

Dr. Sebi believed that people should consume non-GMO foods, as he did with his electrified meals. Fruits and veggies which have been seedless or changed to include more minerals and vitamins than they do organically fall into this category. Dr. Sebi's vegetable list is rather extensive and diversified, giving you dozens of options for creating a variety of tasty meals.

This list contains the following items:

- Amaranth greens, popularly known as Callaloo, are a Kale variation.
- Avocado
- Peppers (bell)
- Mexican Squash – (Chayote)
- Cucumbers
- Greens (Dandelion)
- Garbanzo beans of Garbanzo
- Bananas, green
- Flower/ leaf of cactus - (Izote)
- Kale
- Lettuce (excluding Iceberg)
- Mushrooms of all kinds (excluding Shiitake)
- Mexican Cactus – (Nopales)
- Okra
- Olives (not drenched in vinegar)
- Onions
- Greens in a poke salad
- Purslane (Verdolaga)
- Sea veggies (Wakame/ arame/ nori and etc)
- Squash, except for pumpkin
- Tomatoes (just cherry & plum/Roma)
- Tomatillo
- Greens from turnips
- Watercress
- Zucchini

Fruits

Whereas the vegetable inventory is very extensive, the fruit selection is more limited, with several fruits being prohibited on the Dr. Sebi diet. On the other hand, the list of the fruit continues to provide a varied range of alternatives for diet adherents. For example, all berry kinds are permitted on the Dr. Sebi dietary list, except for cranberries, which seem to be a man-made fruit. In addition, the following items are also on the list:

(No packaged or seedless fruits are allowed.)

- Apples
- Bananas
- Berries of all kinds (excluding cranberries)
- Cantaloupe
- Dates
- Figs
- Seeded grapes
- Limes
- Mango
- Seeded melons
- Orange
- Papayas
- Peaches
- Pear
- Plums
- Pear Prickly (Cactus Fruit)
- Prune
- Seeded Raisins
- Soursops
- Tamarind

Grains

- Amaranth
- Fonio
- Kamut
- Quinoa

- Rye
- Spelt
- Teff
- Rice (Wild)

Nuts and Seeds

- Seeds of hemp
- Sesame seeds, uncooked
- Tahini butter/raw sesame seeds

- Walnuts
- Brazil nuts

Oils

- Coconut oil (unprocessed)
- Olive oil (unprocessed)
- Avocado oil
- Oil made from grape-seeds

- Oil made from hempseed
- Oil extracted from sesame seed

Spices and Seasonings

- Bay leaf
- Cloves

- Basil
- Dill

- Oregano
- Parsley
- Savory
- Sweet basil
- Tarragon
- Thyme
- Sea Salt (Pure)

- Finely ground Coarse Seaweed
- Agave Syrup
- Achiote
- Coriander (Cilantro)
- Habanero
- Powdered onion

What Is Mucus and Its Relation to Different Diseases

What is mucus?

Mucus is a preventive substance secreted from the mouth, nose, throat, lungs, stomach, and intestines, among other areas. Mucus is made up of many different components, but the most important is a molecule called mucin. Based on their structure, mucins in mucus may act as a physical barrier, lubricating content, or viscous substance. Mucus covers surfaces all across our body when its structure and production are normal, allowing us to live alongside various microbes. However, when mucin structure, as well as synthesis, are abnormal, diseases might result.

Mucus is responsible for more than just congestion. It is very good for our health since it traps pathogens and protects the body from infections.

Dr. Sebi remarked, "Mucus is the source of all diseases," "Get rid of the mucus, and you'll get rid of the sickness." Dr. Sebi claimed mucus & acidity induced illness.

According to experts, variations in the type and amount of mucus may contribute to suffering in several chronic conditions. However, the sticky substance that lines our lungs, digestive tracts, and other sections of our bodies is, for the most being, a symptom of the problem rather than a cause.

However, if an improper quantity of mucus is present, it can make things difficult. The quantity of mucus required is comparable to the 'Three Bears' concept, in which too much and too little is a problem, and it must be exactly perfect. For the most being, excessive mucus is a side effect of being unwell, such as when you have a cough and a runny nose. It is not the primary cause of disease. Mucus irregularities or overproduction, on the other hand, may lead to illness in specific cases.

Abnormal mucus is a pathological aspect of some disorders, like asthma and cystic fibrosis, and it leads to disease. For example, too much mucus builds up in cystic fibrosis, a genetic illness that impairs mucus production all across the body, and chronic bronchitis, a lung infection in which bacteria thrive. Every day, the average human produces more than a liter of mucus. This comprises snot, saliva, cervical mucus, and digestive, urinary, pulmonary, nasal, and protective eye layers.

Excessive Mucus Production: Causes & Risk Factors

Excessive mucus, also known as excess sputum, is a symptom of several chronic respiratory disorders, acute infections, and environmental irritants. Some varieties of COPD (chronic obstructive pulmonary disease), for example, are characterized by excessive mucus production and a reduced capacity to filter mucus from the lungs.

Mucus is frequently confused with saliva. However, the two are not quite the same. Saliva is a liquid generated in the mouth that aids in digestion and swallowing meals. Mucus traps dead cells & detritus from the respiratory tracts, allowing it (along with any organisms, like bacteria) to be ponied up and out of the lungs.

While this is good for your body, excessive mucus production, especially unclaimed and continuous, may lead to respiratory problems and a high chance of infection.

The Most Common Causes

Excessive sputum may be present all of the time with several chronic respiratory disorders. At times, you may have severe flare-ups with considerably more sputum than normal. Even if your lungs are in good condition, you may have excessive sputum throughout a respiratory disease. Goblet cells, as well as sub-mucosal glands, create mucus. Failure of these cells, infection, swelling, irritation or residue in the respiratory tract may cause overproduction or hyper-secretion.

Smoking and some medical diseases may cause damage to the cilia, which are microscopic hair-like structures that assist the transport of mucus out of the lungs. Coughing ability may also be hampered by atrophy (shrinkage) of the muscles involved in coughing. Excessive respiratory mucus is usually associated with the following conditions:

Infection of the lungs

Anyone may have a short-term respiratory disease that causes mucus to build up in the lungs. A minor bacterial or viral respiratory system infection and serious bacterial pneumonia may cause this. Infectious organisms cause the lungs to produce an immune response to clear themselves of the infection. Once you have an illness, your sputum output rises to eliminate invading bacteria. In most cases, the mucus should return to normal following a few days of your recovery.

Asthma

Asthma is characterized by periods of respiratory distress brought on by environmental factors, including airborne particles, pollen, and pet dander. In addition, you might well have hyper mucus secretion throughout an asthma attack.

Bronchitis

Excessive mucus synthesis in the lungs is linked to chronic bronchitis, a kind of COPD. Therefore, coughing with sputum production daily for a minimum of three months is one of the diagnostic criteria.

When the situation worsens, the mucus might thicken considerably more than normal.

Emphysema

Emphysema is a kind of COPD characterized by extreme mucus secretion, coughing, and susceptibility to lung infections.

Bronchiectasis

Bronchiectasis is a disorder in which recurring infections cause the airways to enlarge permanently. As a result, Bronchiectasis causes thick, foul-smelling sputum to be produced.

Edema of the lungs

A hazardous rise in lung fluid may occur due to pulmonary edema. Sputum is frequently frothy and maybe pink in color, attributed to the existence of blood.

Genetics

Increased mucus is linked to several genetic illnesses. Some illnesses directly impact the lungs, whereas others wreak havoc on the muscles that control breathing, increasing respiratory mucus.

Cystic fibrosis is a hereditary condition that affects the respiratory and gastrointestinal systems, among other bodily systems. One of the most distinguishing features of this illness is increased mucus production.

Primary ciliary dyskinesia is a hereditary illness characterized by faulty cilia, resulting in excessive mucus in the lungs and susceptibility to infections and breathing problems.

Excess mucus may also be caused by neuromuscular diseases, including muscular dystrophy and spinal muscular atrophy, which impede muscle function and diminish lung movement during inhaling and exhaling, as well as your strength and capacity to cough. Mucus accumulates in the lower lung as a result of this.

Chapter 3: Detoxification and Cleansing

What is Detoxification?

Detoxification is a naturally occurring phenomenon in our bodies that eliminate and convert toxins and undesirable elements. It is our body's major function, and it continually functions and integrates with the remaining body's functions. As a result, it is a mechanism that maintains our bodies healthy and enhances and optimizes their performance. This is accomplished by reducing the toxins we introduce into the body and simultaneously providing the body's removal and detoxification processes with the nutrients they need to function properly.

The liver is where detoxification begins. Your liver basically achieves this in two steps, although it's a difficult procedure. First, toxic chemicals are converted to highly reactive metabolites, eventually excreted. Second, detoxification is supported by the kidneys, lungs, or even the gut. Toxins may have an immediate and long-term effect on these organs. The long-lasting, low-grade toxins found in commercially farmed fruits and vegetables are more harmful, such as residue. Because reactions aren't instantaneous, you can overlook the link between persistent low-grade toxins and weight loss struggles.

Although the detoxification process is the most neglected by today's healthcare system, it is an important element of functioning. The majority of the molecules produced in our bodies daily are used to eliminate waste products. The body needs hundreds of enzymes, vitamins, and many other compounds to help it eliminate waste and toxins. We need to make these molecules to help us focus on the good according to what we eat and leave the harmful. However, the liver, along with the digestive tract, does the majority of the job; the kidneys, lymph system, lungs, and skin are all engaged in the complicated system of detoxification.

The major goal of detoxification systems is to assist the organs and digest and eliminate the toxins in the human body. So it's necessary for optimal health.

What exactly does a full-body detox entail?

A whole-body detox is a method that some individuals think may help them get rid of toxins. It might include following a certain diet, fasting, supplementing, or utilizing a sauna.

Detoxes may promote healthier habits like eating a balanced diet, exercising regularly, and being hydrated, which can help the body's natural detoxification mechanisms. A complete body detox, often known as cleansing, is a program individuals undertake to rid their bodies of toxins. Toxins are chemicals that harm one's health, like poisons and pollutants. The liver, kidneys, gastrointestinal system, and skin are all capable of removing these chemicals on their own.

There is no one-size-fits-all explanation of what a full-body detox entails, although it may entail:

- Stick to a strict diet

- Fast

- Increase your intake of water or juices.

- Make use of supplements

- Utilize laxatives, suppositories, or colonic irrigation

- Use a sauna

- Decrease the exposure to environmental contaminants

There are, however, certain hazards, as well as some detox products that might be dangerous.

How does the detoxification process work?

Detoxification is the process of purifying the blood. This is accomplished by eliminating pollutants from the bloodstream in the liver, which also processes toxins for excretion. Toxins are also eliminated via the kidneys, intestine, lungs, lymphatic vessels, and skin during a physical detox. Impurities aren't effectively filtered when these pathways are weakened, and the body suffers as a result.

A body detox program may assist the natural cleaning process of the body by:

- Fasting to allow the organs to rest

- Helping the liver to eliminate toxins

- Facilitating elimination via the intestine, kidneys, as well as skin

- Boosting blood circulation; and

- Recharging the body with nutritious foods

How do you know if you really need a body detox?

Everybody must detox a minimum of once a year. However, detoxing is not recommended for nursing women, children, or people with chronic degenerative disorders, cancer, or TB. If you're unsure whether or not detox is appropriate for you, talk to your doctor.

"It's vital to detox today," explains Linda Page, N.D., Ph.D., publisher of Detoxification: Strategies to Cleanse, Purify, and Renew, since there are more toxins in the surroundings than ever before.

Detoxing is recommended by Page for symptoms like:

- Fatigue that isn't explained
- Sluggish expulsion
- Irritated skin
- Allergies
- Infection at a low level
- Bags beneath the eyes or puffy eyes
- Bloating
- Menstrual issues
- Mental anguish

What is the best way to begin a body detox?

To begin a physical detox, you'll need to reduce your toxic load first. Remove alcohol, caffeine, cigarettes, refined carbohydrates, and saturated fats from your diet since they all function as poisons in the body and obstruct your recovery. Also, replace natural alternatives for chemical-based home cleaners, including personal health care items (household cleaners, conditioners, deodorants, and toothpaste).

Stress is another barrier to good health since it causes your body to produce stress chemicals into your system. While these hormones might give you an "adrenaline high" to help you win a race or make a deadline, they also generate toxins and shut down the liver's detoxifying enzymes in large doses. Yoga, Qigong, and meditation are all easy and effective strategies to reduce stress by adjusting your physical & mental responses to the stress that life will inevitably bring.

Which detox plan suits you best?

Depending on the specific requirements, there are a variety of detoxification regimens and detox recipes available. However, a 3 to 7-day juice fast (drink only vegetable and fruit juices and water) is recommended by Page as an efficient technique to eliminate toxins.

The following are the top five detox diets:

- Detox with Fruit and Veggies

- Cleanse with a Smoothie

- Cleanse with Juice

- Detox from Sugar

- Detoxification using Hypoallergenic Ingredients

Difference between Detox and Cleansing

While the phrases cleanse and detoxification are often used simultaneously, they are not the same thing! While both eliminate toxins from the body, detoxification or cleanse is not the same! Clean is at the core of the term "cleanse," and you must think of it as a means to clean your body. A cleansing usually focuses on the digestive system and employs supplements or tablets to expel toxins directly. Detox procedures, on either hand, aim to aid your body's natural toxin-removal mechanisms. Because the kidneys and liver are the body's primary detoxifying organs, excellent detox programs involve supporting the liver & kidneys by providing them with the nutrients and supplements they ought to perform at their best.

So, what exactly are toxins?

Heavy metals, such as mercury, are at the forefront. Still, there are also contaminants, plastics, and pesticides on the list. Toxins are hazardous particles that may remain in your body for long periods, aggravating cells, causing inflammation, & interacting with your body's natural activities.

The following are symptoms of toxicity or an extremely toxic load (and consequently the necessity for a detox or cleanse):

- Fatigue

- Headaches

- Joint discomfort

- Depression

- Anxiety

- As well as constipation

The Cleansing Process

Cleansing is linked to maintaining intestinal health. The process of digestion is the system that delivers nutrients to the body. It becomes sluggish in fulfilling its responsibilities if it becomes unwell. An accumulation of waste in the intestines may become poisonous, causing pain and sickness. Bloating is among the symptoms of a sick stomach. Gas builds up whenever the body doesn't even get rid of toxins as quickly as it should. After then, the food starts to decompose. Food ought to be organic and as close to organic as possible.

There are both useful and dangerous bacteria in the digestive system. When the ratio of these microorganisms is disrupted, problems emerge. Purging is by far the most fundamental kind of cleaning. A laxative is used to eliminate wastes, parasites, and other unpleasant substances. However, the difficulty with this technique is that it would be non-selective and eliminate the good along with the bad. It might also be problematic since you can lose too much water in the process, leaving you dehydrated. One of the body's techniques is getting rid of toxic toxins is by drinking enough water.

According to Marie Spano, a nutritionist & vice president of the International Association of Sports Nutrition, exercise and good sleep are crucial to making your cleaning program work for you.

It's a good idea to start the cleaning process by mending the gut by watching what passes into it. Unhealthy food is so termed because it lacks the body's minerals to function properly. Instead, it clogs the digestive system, causing it to malfunction. Gluten, soy, fructose, dairy, and caffeine-containing foods should be avoided and substituted with organic, additive-free alternatives.

The cleansing process does not end with removing waste from the digestive system. Instead, it must be repaired by supplying nutritious food that helps the intestines function optimally. This includes fiber-rich, nutritious foods that aid in restoring adequate levels of organisms, such as beneficial bacteria in the gut. Natural beverages, including unflavored probiotic yogurt, may also help.

To begin the cleaning regimen, you must have been through a pre-cleanse period in which you must abstain from drinking alcohol and eating various harmful foods. Therefore, the first few days in the program were difficult. However, when the body adapted and began to work better, a significant increase in overall energy levels can be seen.

The Detox Technique

Detoxification is another method of removing hazardous substances from the body. Toxins are normally eliminated from the body via the skin, liver, and kidneys. Detox is intended to help these organs work more efficiently. So, which toxins are the procedure aimed at? For one thing, the oxygen you breathe contains toxins that make their way into the body and cause irritation. In addition, pesticides, preservatives, and flavors are all found in a lot of food.

Gwyneth Paltrow is among the celebs that have found success with detox. It takes place over 21 days. The Clean Program is the name given to it by the doctor who created it. To get rid of pollutants, he recommends a diet of smoothies, clean meals, plus supplements. The majority of the patients say they lost weight due to the approach.

Your skin is also exposed to a toxic cocktail contained in the creams, lotions, and other products you use. As a result, the organs in charge of detoxification might sometimes get overworked.

Cleanse the Body Naturally with Food

The essential technique to detox is to eat a balanced diet. To begin, eliminate foods that obstruct detoxification or leave you highly toxic. Fructose, which is present in soda (as high-fructose syrup of corn or HFCS) and fruit juices & commercialized juice cleanses, is one of them. According to research, this simple sugar might have a role in chronic disorders, including obesity. Fructose increases persistent inflammation and oxidative stress, both of which lead to obesity.

Reducing Tran's fats and degraded fats is also part of natural cleansing. Even though the front label reads "low in fat," these fats may be found in processed goods that have "partially hydrogenated" in the components. Damaged fats, such as poached eggs on the banquet table, have been damaged and should be avoided.

Food allergies may impede weight loss and aggravate toxicity by rendering your gut more porous and enabling toxins to access the bloodstream. Common food sensitivities include gluten, milk products, soy, and corn. Try avoiding these meals if you're thinking of detoxing your body.

"The reasonable strategy is to use a focus on food to assist the incredibly complicated mechanisms of detoxification and biotransformation," says John Cline, MD. "It's preferable to consume an apple as part of a range of meals than to attempt to imitate its advantages with specific nutritional supplements if an apple includes at least 700 distinct phytochemicals."

The Safest Foods for Detoxification

Oils and Fats

Olive oil and organic coconut oil are natural fats and oils that give energy for the detoxification and biotransformation mechanisms.

Seeds & Nuts

For a nutritious snack, try Brazilian nuts, walnuts, as well as hempseeds. Nuts & seeds are high in fiber, which helps with normal excretion and elimination.

Proteins

Protein is required to efficiently function the two primary detoxification routes found inside the liver cells, known as Phase 1 & Phase 2. So, again, organic grass-fed cattle and wild-caught fish are the best choices.

Legumes

Insoluble and soluble fiber, and a spectrum of amino acid precursors, may be found in beans, lentils, and other legumes.

Fruits

Fruits include a range of phytonutrients with antioxidant qualities, like beta-carotene, lutein, & anthocyanin's. They're also rich in water and an excellent source of soluble & insoluble fiber.

Vegetables

Non-starchy veggies are high in phytochemicals and fiber, among other nutrients.

A body-cleanse diet consists mostly of nutrient-dense, low-sugar, high-fiber plant-based foods and high-protein and healthy nutrition fat sources. Most food products, especially inflammatory fats, would be eliminated in favor of whole, unadulterated, natural foods.

Consume organic plant foods wherever feasible. According to the Environmental Working Group, normal food includes 178 pesticides. If organic isn't an option due to cost or availability, consult the EWG's list of the most — & least — pesticide-laden fruits and vegetables, labeled the Dirty Dozen as well as Clean 15, respectively.

Food contains nutrients that aid in detoxification, but therapeutic amounts of particular nutrients may also effectively cleanse the liver and other detoxifying organs naturally. Therefore, a complete variety of nutrients to promote liver function and detoxification should be tailored to the individual's requirements.

Chiropractors assist patients in selecting the proper nutrients ineffective levels to detoxify daily. A chiropractor or even other physicians may also create a personalized detoxification approach for you that incorporates a healthy diet.

10 Natural Techniques to Aid Your Body's Detoxification Process

Make regular detox a priority to promote liver health and the body's natural detoxification processes so you may achieve (and remain) lean, healthy, as well as enthusiastic while lowering your disease susceptibility. Here are some methods for getting rid of toxins.

2. Consume the appropriate meals

Numerous studies have shown that whole foods like green vegetables, berries, and seasonings like turmeric might assist detoxification in numerous ways. When combined with protein and good fat, these whole foods form an ideal detox and weight-loss diet.

2. Trust your gut.

GI Renew is a supplement that replenishes intestinal flora.

A dysfunctional detoxification system is caused or exacerbated by gastrointestinal disorders. Therefore, optimizing the digestive system necessitates reducing the impediments that cause dysbiosis (gut abnormalities) and other issues and consuming the right gut-supporting foods and minerals.

See your chiropractor and other health professionals if you anticipate intestinal permeability (leaking gut) or other digestive issues.

3. Lower the level of inflammation

Toxicity causes inflammation, which leads to a higher toxic load and, as a result, fat loss is hindered. Wild-caught fish, omega-3-rich plant foods like flaxseed & chia seeds, non-starchy veggies, and spices like turmeric are all part of an anti-inflammatory diet. Integrate anti-inflammatory ingredients such as fish oil, oil of krill, resveratrol, as well as curcumin into the diet with the help of your chiropractor and other healthcare providers.

4. Maintain a healthy immune system

At the very least, make sure you eat properly, get enough sleep, control your stress, practice appropriate hygiene, such as hand washing, and receive adequate nutrients to promote healthy immunity.

5. Increase the effectiveness of your natural detoxification process.

While the cells are continually detoxing, consider undergoing a full-body detox in the spring (or autumn). These two- to three-week regimens contain everything you need to help your liver and other organs detox properly, such as protein, minerals, and a detox-minded food plan.

6. Keep your exposure to a minimum

The first line of defense is always prevention on offense and defense. Toxins may be found in home cleaners, construction materials, plastic, junk foods, and other sources. The Environmental Working Group (EWG) is a wonderful place to start since it has various information, including how to detect toxins in your life.

7. Drink lots of water that is free of contaminants

Hydration maintains your cellular machinery working smoothly, allowing it to cleanse and perform various other activities. To prevent additional contaminants, use water that has been adequately filtered.

8. Wipe the toxins out

Exercise has a range of benefits, including assisting the body better, eliminating toxins & burning fat. Find a regular fitness routine that matches your preferences and schedule, whether it's hot yoga as well as high-intensity interval training.

9. Have plenty of rest

A few years ago, researchers discovered the glymphatic system, a brain detoxification mechanism that happens when you sleep. Insufficient sleep, as per Andy R. Eugene and Jolanta Masiak, causes toxin build-up by impairing the glymphatic system. The body cannot adequately detoxify if you do not get enough decent sleep in the necessary proportions regularly.

10. Make an appointment with a chiropractor

The neurological system, which governs all metabolic routes, such as detoxification pathways, is affected by chiropractic adjustments. Adjusting your perspective will allow your body to cleanse and operate at its best. Toxic overload is a common cause of obesity. The correct detoxification plan may supply your body with the nutrients it needs to repair and lose weight. While these tactics are a fine place to begin, a chiropractor and another healthcare expert can help you create a detoxification strategy suited to your specific needs.

Detoxification Through Fasting

Fasting throughout Ramadan is directed in Islam, but it is both curative and preventative for several of the diseases that individuals suffer from due to poor eating and living patterns. Fasting was suggested by traditional healers hundreds of years ago due to the outstanding health advantages of willingly giving up meals and drinks for extended periods. However, fasting is perhaps the most important natural healing remedy unavailable in today's Western culture. The recent rise of affluent disorders like atherosclerosis, hypertension, cardiovascular disease, infections, diabetes, and cancer may be linked to the abandonment of this age-old practice in the West.

These ailments are becoming increasingly widespread in Muslim communities as well, resulting from not fasting appropriately and deviating from the original aim of fasting.

For centuries, fasting has been adopted in Jews, Christians, Islam, and Eastern cultures as a therapeutic, spiritual, religious, and cleansing procedure. In addition, fasting therapy has been employed and believed in by Socrates, Plato, Aristotle, and Hippocrates to restore health where there was disease.

Fasting's therapeutic properties are since it is a sort of detoxification from gluttony and susceptibility of our bodies to harmful substances in our diet and surroundings. But, of course, we can't live in bubbles to shield our bodies from these pollutants. Still, we can use fasting properly to benefit from its cleansing benefits.

Detoxification is a popular and trendy term, but what exactly does it imply? Detoxification is the procedure of lowering toxins' intake and expelling them from the body or changing them & eliminating excessive mucus and congestion to restore the body's natural functioning and healing abilities.

Nicotine and other dangerous medications, air pollution, lipids, cholesterol, even free radicals are all examples of toxins. Fasting promotes excretion processes and increases the discharge of pollutants from the colon, kidneys, bladder, and the lungs & respiratory system, sinuses, and skin. In addition, we enable the digestive tract to rest by not constantly eating throughout the day.

By reducing the amount of effort required for the digestive organs, such as the intestine, stomachs, liver, gallbladder, pancreas, as well as the kidneys, to heal and restore themselves, eliminate underlying toxins, and mop up the flowing blood & lymph, the body can heal and restore itself. The body expends a lot of energy in the process of breaking down meals. The energy that would typically be spent on digestion is now offloaded and may be utilized to improve health and vitality, as well as enhance mental abilities

Fasting may help with a variety of health issues. For example, indigestion, impaired bowel function, and extra belly fat put pressure on the back muscles, leading to a variety of back problems. Fasting and a reduced diet in the evenings may help with this sort of back pain. In addition, allergies & sinus congestion may be alleviated by fasting, which helps the body clear itself of extra mucus.

- Weight reduction may be achieved throughout the month of Ramadan as long as people do not overindulge in meals and desserts after the fast is completed.

- Fasting is an effective way to break coffee, cigarettes, and even narcotics addictions.

- Fasting for 5 to 7 days will greatly diminish the intense desire for hazardous drugs.

- Fasting is a powerful motivation to break unhealthy habits and a catalyst for transformation and personal development.

Fasting is a great approach to cleanse, particularly if you can eat fruits & light veggies throughout your fasting routine. The list of items to avoid throughout a detox program is almost identical to shun during a fast. The key is to consume light, fresh, and unprocessed food. This may differ based on people's beliefs and practices. However, that's precisely what a detox suggests as well.

Consider the fact that the human body detoxes naturally daily. For example, the digestive system removes undigested food while the lungs expel carbon dioxide-rich air. The skin, too, uses pores and sweat glands to remove waste and perspiration. Besides these natural detox mechanisms, the body may need extra assistance in eliminating toxins accumulated over time.

How Frequently Should You Do It?

Excessive mucus, food scraps, sludge, old feces, and artificial mineral deposits may all be removed with a 3- to 7-day detox. Even a quick fast removes toxins from the body. While fasting may be a fantastic method to cleanse and reset your system, it's critical to make sure the water you're drinking has a high nutritional content.

Fasting with water:

Fasting with water has been and remains to be among the most powerful healing methods in history. There are several debates on water fasting by prominent ancient figures such as Plato, Aristotle, Socrates, Leonardo Da Vinci, and Pythagoras. Furthermore, there is a variety of fresh material on water fasting accessible on the Internet, which may assist in self-education about the various methods of fasting and the advantages of fasting.

Scientific studies have shown that your brain actually develops when you fast, and you'll be cleverer. Furthermore, according to recent research, three-day water fast resets your immune function by stimulating stem cells, allowing you to function at your best. Every day, we perform a range of activities, such as breathing contaminated air, and drink tainted beverages, and so on, clogging the body filters, including the lungs, mouth, liver, as well as kidneys. Human bodies heat up with time, and indeed the immune system suffers as a result. Fevers cause the body to sweat off toxins and generate a natural fasting response. In such situations, three-to-four-day water fast is beneficial. This will aid in the cleansing of your system. So, should you simply let the body go through the biological cycle of being really ill and in agony to properly cleanse the system? There's no need to become ill if you clean the cleaners constantly by conducting water fast.

Intermittent fasting is a more convenient alternative to complete water fast. Essentially, you don't eat anything at all for one day in a week, allowing the kidneys and liver to properly detoxify and eliminate any pollutants. It is, however, critical to properly hydrate oneself throughout those 24 hours, either via drinking enough water or through other means. You may also take a salt flush, an evacuation, breathing techniques, and natural skin washing to help flush out the toxins.

Fasting is frequently discouraged for diabetics and hypoglycemics. Still, it might possibly help human bodies discharge stem cells and restore themselves with the correct assistance. For example, you may begin an intermittent fast at noon, skip supper, sleep, skip breakfast, and resume eating at lunch break. This is among the simplest methods, and providing you remain well hydrated; you should have no difficulty. If you can't commit to the whole 24 hours, omitting a small meal may be helpful.

Fasting on juice:

A juice cleanses a form of detox diet that entails drinking only vegetable and fruit juice for a certain time (typically 1 to 3 days). Some plans incorporate one or even more smoothies each day to deliver energy and hunger relief by providing protein, fat, and other nutrients. On certain plans, vegan meals, as well as snacks, are provided.

A juice cleanses, according to supporters, aids the body's natural detoxification processes, purifies the diet of sweets, caffeine, processed meats, and other foods and chemicals that diminish energy, & jumpstarts a healthier eating pattern.

Because the nutrients, phytochemicals, and antioxidants are in a readily absorbable liquid form, unfiltered organic juice is a major component of the cleansing. For those who require more energy, are a novice to juice cleanses, or prefer a less severe experience, vegan, gluten-free snacks and meals may be included. A juicer/juice press may be used to do a juice detox at home.

Chapter 4: 28-Day Detox Plan

Tiredness, exhaustion, weight gain, sleep problems, thyroid problems, reduced libido, digestive problems, a loss of mojo, despair, anxiety, eczema, and addictions are symptoms that your body needs to detox.

Getting rid of toxins

Keeping the colon and lymphatic systems more effective is a significant aspect of the detox because it allows them to start clearing out the ama (digestive toxins from unprocessed food & muck in the system) through the main detoxification. To do so, you'll need to free up the paths via the kidneys; blocked pipes can't be flushed out. You'll also be passing items through the colon more quickly while supporting your gut flora's garden.

How Are The 28 Days Divided?

The first phase, which lasts from day 1 to day 14: is all about removing toxins from your diet and lifestyle so that your body can prepare for what's ahead. A full-time fasting is required. No food nor liquid (except water) is allowed.

The second phase goes from day 15 to day 28: the moment to truly build on the success you've achieved in the previous stage, which is the past 14 days. In this phase you should aim to drink 3-4 different alkaline smoothies each day, selecting the recipes from the ones below.

Days	Breakfast	Lunch	Dinner
1	Water + Herbal Teas	Water + Herbal Teas	Water + Herbal Teas
2	Water + Herbal Teas	Water + Herbal Teas	Water + Herbal Teas
3	Water + Herbal Teas	Water + Herbal Teas	Water + Herbal Teas
4	Water + Herbal Teas	Water + Herbal Teas	Water + Herbal Teas
5	Water + Herbal Teas	Water + Herbal Teas	Water + Herbal Teas
6	Water + Herbal Teas	Water + Herbal Teas	Water + Herbal Teas
7	Water + Herbal Teas	Water + Herbal Teas	Water + Herbal Teas
8	Water + Herbal Teas	Water + Herbal Teas	Water + Herbal Teas
9	Water + Herbal Teas	Water + Herbal Teas	Water + Herbal Teas
10	Water + Herbal Teas	Water + Herbal Teas	Water + Herbal Teas
11	Water + Herbal Teas	Water + Herbal Teas	Water + Herbal Teas
12	Water + Herbal Teas	Water + Herbal Teas	Water + Herbal Teas
13	Water + Herbal Teas	Water + Herbal Teas	Water + Herbal Teas
14	Water + Herbal Teas	Water + Herbal Teas	Water + Herbal Teas
15	Alkaline Shake Post-Workout	Smoothie with Kale	Blueberry-Banana Smoothie
16	Smoothie with Kiwi & Cucumber	Turmeric Ginger Citrus	Berry Smoothie
17	Super-simple Watermelon Juice	Blueberry Alkaline Smoothie	Vegetable Punch

18	Apple-Ginger Smoothie	Super Smoothie with Kale and Strawberry	Apple-Ginger Smoothie
19	Hempseed Milk Alkaline Smoothie	Kiwi Alkaline Smoothie	Flax Seeds Alkaline Smoothie
20	Blueberry Alkaline Smoothie	Smoothie with Grapefruit	Detox Juice
21	Turmeric Ginger Citrus	Vegetable Punch	Orange Sunrise Mix
22	Detox Juice	Romain Lettuce and Grapefruit Smoothie	Hempseed Milk Alkaline Smoothie
23	Super-simple Watermelon Juice	Kiwi Alkaline Smoothie	Berry Smoothie
24	Vegetable Punch	Green Alkaline Smoothie	Apple-Ginger Smoothie
25	Green Juice	Flax Seeds Alkaline Smoothie	Turmeric Ginger Citrus
26	Blueberry-Banana Smoothie	Turmeric Ginger Citrus	Hempseed Milk Alkaline Smoothie
27	Orange Sunrise Mix	Vegetable Punch	Blueberry Alkaline Smoothie
28	Green Alkaline Smoothie	Super Smoothie with Kale and Strawberry	Detox Juice

Chapter 5: Juice and Smoothie Recipes

1. Hempseed Milk Alkaline Smoothie

Ingredients

- 1 cup hempseed milk
- 1 cup diced watermelon
- 5 strawberries (fresh or iced)
- 1/2 of a tiny banana
- 1 cup of kale
- 1 tsp. chia seeds
- 1 cup ice

Directions

- Combine the kale, tiny banana, chia seeds, half of the ice, and half of the hempseed milk in a blender. Blend until everything is properly incorporated.
- Blend in the remaining milk & ice with the watermelon and iced strawberries.
- Dump in the smoothie and stir until fully mixed.

2. Kiwi Alkaline Smoothie

Ingredients

- 1/4 cup coconut milk
- 1/4 cup of cucumber
- 1/2 of a banana
- 1 kiwi
- 1 cup of kale
- 4 or 5 ice cubes

Directions

- Bring all of the ingredients together.
- Combine the coconut milk, 1/4 cucumber, banana, kiwi, and kale in a blender and blend until smooth.
- Chill before serving.

3. Green Avocado Smoothie

Ingredients

- 1 pitted and scraped avocado
- 1 cup hempseed milk
- 1 lime's juice
- 1 tsp. cinnamon
- 2 kale leaves

- A few pieces of cucumber

Directions

- Combine all of the ingredients in a blender, and enjoy!

4. Smoothie with Grapefruit

Ingredients

- 1 grapefruit
- 1 cup of coconut milk
- 1 cup of kale
- 1 tsp. organic agave nectar – for sweetness

Directions

- Combine all of the ingredients in a blender, then serve and enjoy!

5. Romain Lettuce and Grapefruit Smoothie

Ingredients

- 2 grapefruits
- 1 head of romaine lettuce
- 1 cup of coconut water
- 1/2 cup pomegranate pits
- ½ cup of alkaline water

Directions

- Deseed, then peel the grapefruit.

- Romain lettuce should be washed and clean.

- Blend all of the components together until they make a creamy, foamy texture. Sweeten with the organic agave nectar.

6. Smoothie with Strawberries

Ingredients

- 2 cups of kale
- ½ cup strawberries
- 1 lime's juice
- 1 banana
- 1 cup coconut water
- 1 tsp. hemp seeds

Directions

- In a blender, combine all ingredients and mix until creamy & frothy.

- To sweeten the smoothie, if necessary, add some organic agave nectar.

7. Smoothie with Kale

Ingredients

- 1 cup kale
- 1 banana
- ½ strawberries

- 1/4 cup raspberries
- 1 cup organic orange juice

Directions

- Fresh as well as frozen berries and bananas may be used.
- Combine all of the ingredients in a blender and blend until smooth.
- If you would like to be more invigorating, add ice if it's a hot day. Enjoy!

8. Green Alkaline Smoothie

Ingredients

- 2 cups of kale
- ½ cup of romaine lettuce
- 1 cup of apple juice
- 1 tbsp. lime juice
- 1/2 cucumber
- ½ cup of coconut water

Directions

- Take a couple of fistful of kale, 1/2 medium cucumber, 1 cup of apple juice, and 1 tablespoon fresh lime juice.
- In a blender, combine all of these ingredients until smooth. Serve and have fun.

9. Flax Seeds Alkaline Smoothie

Ingredients

- 1 tbsp. flaxseeds
- 1 cup of kale
- ½ cup of strawberries
- 1 tsp. of cinnamon
- 1 banana
- 1 tsp. of ginger
- 1 cup of coconut water

Directions

- Combine all of the ingredients in a blender and mix until smooth. Serve and enjoy your drink.
- You may substitute any sort of fruit to replace the strawberries and kale rather than kale.

10. Blueberry Alkaline Smoothie

Ingredients

- ½ cup of blueberries
- 1 cup of kale
- 1 tbsp. of chia seeds
- 1 tbsp. of flaxseeds, ground
- 1 cup of coconut milk
- 1 tbsp. of coconut oil

- 1 tablespoon of hemp seed

Directions

- Simply combine all of the ingredients in a blender and mix until smooth.

- Hemp milk may be substituted with coconut milk if desired.

11. Alkaline Peach & Kale Smoothie

Ingredients

- ¼ cup of peaches
- 1 cup of kale
- 1/2 cucumber
- 1/4 cup of parsley
- 1 banana
- 1/2 cup water
- 1/2 of a lime's juice

Directions

- Peaches should be sliced and blended.

- In a blender, combine the other ingredients, mix until smooth, and serve.

12. Berry Smoothie

Ingredients

- ½ cup of blueberries
- 1 lime's juice

- 1 tbsp. of chia seeds
- ½ cup of strawberries
- 1 cup of kale
- 1 tsp. of cinnamon
- ½ of a banana
- 1 cup of coconut water

Directions

- In a blender, combine all of the ingredients.

- Fresh or frozen berries may be used.

- You may drink it straight from the blender or mix it with ice for a more delicious drink.

13. Veggie Blast Smoothie

Ingredients

- 1 cucumber, trimmed and chopped
- 4 flaked tomatoes
- 1/2 onion
- 1/2 cup of chilled rosemary infusion
- 1 tablespoon of extra-virgin olive oil
- 1 cup of kale or kale juice
- 1 lime's juice

- ½ cup of coconut water

Directions

- Place the kale and lime juice in a large bowl and put them aside.

- Combine the cucumber, peeled tomatoes, clove, onion, rosemary infusion, and olive oil. Then combine them with kale as well as lime juice in a blender.

- Lastly, season with salt and pepper. Serve immediately this insanely healthy and tasty smoothie.

14. Kale and Fruit Blast Smoothie

Ingredients

- 2 scraped and cored apples

- 1 flaked mango, cut into pieces

- 1 banana

- 1 tbsp. of lime juice

- 1 tiny ginger slice – to taste

- 2 cups of water

- 1 cup of kale

- 2 strands of parsley

Directions

In a blender, combine all ingredients until they form a foamy texture. Serve and have fun.

15. Super Smoothie with Kale and Strawberry

Ingredients

- 2 cups of kale

- 1/2 cup strawberry

- 1 lime

- 1 banana

- 1 cup of coconut water

- 1 tbsp. of hemp seeds

Directions

- In a blender, combine all ingredients and mix until smooth.

- It's worth noting that the banana might be fresh or frozen. Instead of putting the entire lime in the blender, squeeze out the juice. Even though the smoothie will most likely be sweet already, you may sweeten it with organic agave nectar.

16. Smoothie with Kiwi and Cucumber

Ingredients

- 1 kiwi

- 1/4 cucumber

- 1/2 banana

- 1 handful of kale

- ½ cup coconut milk

Directions

- Put all of the ingredients in a blender and mix until smooth. Put a few ice cubes into the blender if you really want to make the smoothie even more refreshing.

17. Alkaline Breakfast Smoothie

Ingredients

- 2 grapefruits

- 2 heads of romaine lettuce

- 1/2 cup arils of pomegranate

- 1 cup of coconut water

Directions

- The grapefruits must first be peeled and the seeds removed

- Combine the ingredients in a blender. For sweetness, you may also want to add 1 tsp. of organic agave nectar.

18. Smoothie with Alkaline Energy Boosters

Ingredients

- 1 cup of kale

- 1 banana

- 1/2 cup strawberry

- 1 cup of orange juice

- 1/4 cup of raspberries

Directions

- You may use fresh or frozen raspberries, strawberries, as well as bananas. In a blender, combine the ingredients and add several ice cubes to keep it more refreshing.

19. Smoothie with Alkaline Greens

Ingredients

- 2 handfuls of kale

- 1 cup of apple juice

- 1 tbsp. freshly squeezed lime juice

- 1/2 cucumber

Directions

- Combine all of the ingredients in a blender and mix until smooth.

20. Alkaline Smoothie with Extraordaberries

Ingredients

- ½ cup of blueberries
- 1 lime juice
- 1 tbsp. of chia seeds
- 1/2 cup of strawberry
- 1 handful of kale
- 1 tsp. of cinnamon
- 1/2 banana
- 1 cup of coconut water

Directions

- Squeeze the lime into the processor and combine it with the other components.

21. Alkaline Shake Post-Workout

Ingredients

- 1 avocado
- 1 cup of coconut milk
- 1 banana
- 1 tbsp. of chia seeds

Directions

- Combine all of the ingredients in a blender and mix until smooth.

22. Alkaline Smoothie with Peaches and Kale

Ingredients

- ¼ cup of peaches
- 1 cup of kale
- 1/2 cucumbers
- 1/4 cup of parsley
- 1 banana
- 1/2 cup of water
- 1/2 lime juice

Directions

- Squeeze approximately half of a medium-sized lime into a cup. Before placing the peaches in the processor, make sure they're sliced. Then, blend everything together with a couple of ice cubes.

23. Alkaline Smoothie with Blueberries

Ingredients

- ½ of blueberries
- 1 handful of kale
- 1 tbsp. of chia seeds
- 1 tbsp. of flax seeds
- 1 cup of coconut milk

- 1 tbsp. of coconut oil
- 1 tbsp. of hemp seed

Directions

- Simply combine the ingredients in a blender, and your smoothie is ready. Depending on your preferences, you may substitute hemp milk for coconut milk.

24. Alkaline Smoothie with Anti-Inflammatory Properties

Ingredients

- 1 tbsp. of flaxseed
- 1 cup of kale
- 1/2 cup of strawberries
- 1 tsp. of cinnamon
- 1 banana
- 1 tsp. of ginger powder
- 1 cup of coconut water

Directions

- Blend together all of the components until smooth. You may use any sort of berry in place of the strawberries. You may also substitute a handful of kale for the kale.

25. Healthiest Alkaline Juice

Ingredients

- 2 cups of kale
- 1 lime
- 1 pear
- 3 celery stalks
- A handful of fresh parsley
- 1 cup of alkaline water

Directions

- All vegetables should be well cleaned.
- Reduce the size of the pear by chopping it into smaller pieces.
- If you're using a medium juicer, cut the stalks of celery into 1-inch chunks.
- If the lime isn't organic, peel it.
- All of the ingredients should be juiced.
- Stir it well.
- This alkaline juice should be consumed right away. Enjoy.

26. Alkalizing Green Juice

Ingredients

- 1/2 head of Romaine lettuce
- 1 1/2 cup mango, sliced into cubes
- 1 kale leaf, large, coarsely chopped
- 1 lime
- 1 cup of coconut water

Directions

- Thoroughly wash the kale as well as romaine lettuce.
- Mango flesh should be cut into bits. You may also juice the core.
- If you have a centrifugal juicer, you may juice the mango peel.
- If the lime isn't organic, peel it.
- All items should be juiced.

27. Turmeric Ginger Citrus Miracle

Ingredients

- 3 oranges
- 1 lime
- 1-inch slice of ginger
- 1/2 inch chunk of fresh turmeric

Directions

- Remove the peels from the oranges.
- If the lime isn't organic, peel it.
- Peel the turmeric as well as ginger.
- All of the ingredients should be juiced.

28. Super-simple Watermelon Juice

Ingredients

- 1 lime
- 1 tiny sweet watermelon

Directions

- The watermelon should be cut in half.
- If you're using a slow juicer, scoop out the pieces and discard the rind.
- You may juice melon pieces, along with the rind, using a rotating juicer.
- If the lime isn't organic, peel it.
- Everything should be juiced in your juicer.
- Enjoy.

29. Green Juice for Glowing Skin

Ingredients

- 2 apples, peeled and cut into pieces
- 1 cup of kale
- 1 cucumber
- 1 lime juice
- ½ cup of coconut water

Directions

- Rinse the apples, kale, as well as cucumber.
- If the lime & cucumber aren't organic, peel them.
- Using a knife, slice the apple into pieces.
- In a juicer, blend all of the ingredients together.
- Enjoy.

30. Alkalizing Vegetable Juice

Ingredients

- 1 cucumber
- 1 big red pepper
- 1 pear, peeled and cut into pieces
- 1/2 of lime
- ½ cup of alkaline water

Directions

- Everything should be completely cleaned.
- Pare the cucumber and lime.
- In a juicer, blend all of the ingredients together.
- Enjoy.

31. Detox Juice (Alkaline)

Ingredients

- 1 cucumber, medium
- 1 cup coriander
- 1 cup of kale
- 1 apple, peeled and cut into pieces
- 1 lime

Directions

- All vegetables should be well washed.
- Using a knife, slice the apple into pieces.
- If the lime, cucumber, and lime aren't organic, peel them.
- All of the ingredients should be juiced.
- Enjoy the alkaline juice while it's still fresh.

32. Fruit Juice with Alkalizing Properties

Ingredients

- 1 orange
- 2 cups of mango, diced
- 1/2 lime leaves
- ½ cup of alkaline water

Directions

- Remove the peel off the orange
- Remove the skin from the mango and chop it into slices.
- If the lime isn't organic, peel it.
- Everything in the juicer should be juiced

33. Basic Alkaline Juice

Ingredients

- 1 cup coarsely chopped kale
- 1 cucumber, tiny
- 2 cup of mango
- 1 inch of ginger
- 3 celery stalks
- 1 lime
- ½ cup of alkaline water

Directions

- All vegetables should be well washed.
- Chop the kale into small pieces.
- If the ginger, lime, and cucumber aren't organic, peel them.
- Reduce the size of the celery stalks by chopping them into smaller pieces.
- Cut the mango pulp into pieces after removing the skin.
- In a juicer, blend all of the ingredients together.
- Enjoy your alkaline-rich juice.

34. Alkaline Diet Juice

Ingredients

- 2 cups of kale
- 1 cucumber
- 1-inch ginger slice
- 1 lime
- A handful of fresh parsley
- 1 cup of alkaline water

Directions

- Wash all fruits and vegetables thoroughly.

- Pare the cucumber, ginger, as well as lime.

- Everything should be blended in your juicer.

35. Alkalizing Cleanse Juice

Ingredients

- 1 lime
- 1 cup coarsely chopped kale
- 1 piece of cucumber
- 1 cup of kale
- 2 apples, peeled and cut into pieces
- ½ cup of coconut water

Directions

- All vegetables should be well washed.

- Chop the kale into small pieces.

- If the apples, cucumber, and lime are not organic, peel them.

- Chop the apple to fit into the juicer's feed hole.

- Everything within your juice should be blended.

36. Melon Green Juice

Ingredients

- 1/2 melon (honeydew)
- 1 cucumber
- 1 cup of kale
- 1 lime juice
- ½ cup of coconut water

Directions

- Remove the melon's flesh using a fork. The seeds may be juiced.

- If the cucumber isn't organic, peel it, as well as the lime.

- Kale should be washed.

- Everything should be juiced in your juicer.

- This delightful juice should be consumed immediately.

37. Energy Shots with Turmeric and Ginger

Ingredients

- 1/2 inch slice of fresh turmeric
- 1-inch slice of fresh ginger
- 1 lime juice
- ½ cup of hempseed milk

Directions

- If the lime, turmeric root & ginger root aren't organic, peel them.

- End up leaving the peels on if you're blending organic veggies. Simply wash everything completely.

- Everything should be juiced.

- This invigorating turmeric ginger shot is a great way to start your day.

38. Green Smoothie with a Boost

Ingredients

- 2 large leaves of kale
- 1/2 cup diced frozen mango
- 1 banana
- 1 tbsp. lime juice
- 1 cup of alkaline water

Directions

- Place the greens in the processor after thoroughly washing them. Place the mango and a banana in the blender after peeling them. After combining the ingredients, drizzle in the water and combine until smooth.

39. Alkaline Smoothie (Refreshing)

Ingredients

- 1 fistful of fresh kale
- 4 strawberries
- 1 cup diced watermelon
- 1 banana
- 1 cup of coconut milk
- 1 cup of ice cubes

Directions

- Rinse the items before putting them in the processor to juice. If you don't really want a brown smoothie, puree banana, and kale with 1/2 a cup of coconut milk plus ice cubes, then combine the remaining halves with strawberries and watermelon.

- Blend until smooth, then combine the two smoothies in one glass & serve.

40. Alkaline Smoothie with Protein

Ingredients

- 1 avocado
- 1 cup of kale

- 1 banana
- 1 cup of coconut milk

Directions

- You may use a chilled or peeled banana for this recipe. In a blender, combine all of the ingredients and mix until smooth.

41. Juice of Celery

Ingredients

- 1 apple
- 1 celery stem, large (approximately 8 inches long),
- 1/2 of a lime's juice
- 1-inch ginger piece (scraped)
- 1 cucumber
- 1 cup of alkaline water

Directions

- Remove the celery stalks & wash them. Remove any excess water by shaking it off.
- Remove the leaves from the stalks' tops. Place the stalk of celery in the juicer.
- After you've finished with the celery, juice the apple, lime, & ginger.

- It may be consumed immediately away or stored in a small airtight container for three days.

42. Apple-Ginger Juice

Ingredients

- 1 large apple
- 1 tsp. of ginger root, scraped
- 1/4 lime juice
- 1 cup of alkaline water

Directions

- Wash all of your ingredients well and put them aside to cool.
- Toss the lime juice into your cup.
- Toss with ice cubes and a lime slice as a garnish (optional).

43. Vegetable Punch

Ingredients

- 1/2 cup romaine lettuce
- 2 tbsp. of chives, diced
- 1 medium tomato
- ½ of a medium deseeded jalapeno pepper
- 1/2 medium red bell pepper

- 1 celery stalk, large

- ½ cup of coconut water

Directions

- In a juicer, mix the lettuce, chopped chives, tomato, jalapeño, bell pepper, and a stalk of celery

- Serve chilled, adding ice cubes if desired.

- If you don't have a juicer, finely chop all of the ingredients & begin blending with the softer ones first. Blend in the larger and more difficult veggies, lastly. After everything has been mixed, filter the juice through a cheesecloth.

44. Tropical-Kale Delight

Ingredients

- ¼ of a mango

- 1 medium banana

- 1 cup of kale leaves

- ½ cup of coconut water

Directions

- The mango should be cut into strips, and the kale should be coarsely chopped.

- These two should be blended first and then strained. Then,

return the liquid to the processor, along with the banana.

- If you don't mind the chunks from the mango and kale, there's no need to filter the liquid.

45. Orange Sunrise Mix

Ingredients

- 1 large tomato

- 1 medium orange

- 1 large apple

- ½ cup of alkaline water

Directions

- Remove the peel from the orange and wash the rest of the ingredients.

- Cut all fruits and vegetables into bite-sized pieces and place them in the juicer.

- Serve the juice straight up or refrigerate with ice cubes.

46. Green Juice

Ingredients

- 1 ½ cucumbers,

- 1 apple

- A handful of kale

- ½ lime juice

- 1 tsp. of ginger root
- A handful of parsley leaves
- ½ cup of coconut water

Directions

- Clean all of your items well, peel the ginger, and put everything through a blender afterward.

- Pour in half a lime's juice & enjoy.

47. Super Alkaline Cherry Smoothie

Ingredients

- 1 1/2 cup of coconut milk
- 1 cup of seeded fresh cherries
- 1 cup of kale leaves
- 1 kiwi
- 2 tbsp. of walnuts

Directions

- In a high-powered blender, combine all of the ingredients.
- Blend until completely smooth.

48. Blueberry Banana Smoothie

Ingredients

- 1 banana
- ½ cup of blueberries
- Optional: 1/2 tbsp.. ground flaxseed
- Optional: 1/2 tbsp.. hemp seeds
- ½ cup of ice
- ½ cup of vegetable milk of your choice
- 1 cup of alkaline water

Directions

- In a blender, combine the banana, 1/2 cup of blueberries, 1 teaspoon alkaline greens powder, 1/2 tbsp.. Flaxseed, 1/2 tbsp.. Hemp seeds (if utilizing), ice cubes, milk, and water.

- Cover and mix for 1-2 minutes, or until the ingredients are completely processed and smooth.

Chapter 6: Switching From a Standard Diet

The Standard American Diet (SAD) is a contemporary eating pattern with long-term, negative health repercussions for American children and adults. The Standard Diet is defined as high in ultra-processed products, refined sugar, fat, and salt. In addition, this diet is severely low in fruits, veggies, whole grains, legumes, and lean protein.

Making healthy meal choices might seem hard with fast-food chains on virtually every corner as well as fast foods crowding the grocery store shelves. Unfortunately, poor food choices may cause various chronic illnesses, placing pressure on the healthcare system. An overabundance of disinformation in the popular media and a significant lack of awareness among the general people exacerbates the problem. On the other hand, simple dietary modifications may enhance one's health and minimize the chance of acquiring a variety of chronic illnesses.

Switching from standard to alkaline

Shifting to an alkaline diet is the first step on the road to recovery from SAD. Shift to whole foods with high nutritional density instead of highly processed foods like white bread, white rice, and sugary items.

What do you mean by "whole foods"?

Unprocessed foods that are as similar to their original condition as possible, without the need for a tag or a barcode. There are no extra fats, carbohydrates, or artificial additives in these items.

Whole foods offer a higher ratio of vitamins, minerals, and phytonutrients over calories than prepared foods. Plant nutrients are referred to as phytonutrients.

They've been examined extensively for their potential to decrease inflammation and improve overall health. Whole foods like fruit, vegetables, and legumes are the greatest way to receive a variety of phytonutrients.

In conclusion, the path to recovery from SAD starts with diet and lifestyle changes that may also help to reduce inflammation.

The following are some of the protective factors to shift from a standard diet to an Alkaline or plant-based diet:

- Consume greater anti-inflammatory phytonutrients such as carotenoids and bioflavonoids-rich fruits and veggies.

- Consume sufficient omega-3 fatty acids, such as those found in fish, flaxseed, green vegetables, as well as sea vegetables.

- Increasing the amount of fiber consumed.

- 30 - 60 min of mild to intense aerobic exercise each day

- Eliminate your consumption of ultra-processed meals

- Fruits and vegetables should be prioritized

- Increase your intake of plant-based proteins

- Half of your grains should be whole

- Sugar additives must be avoided

- Make more meals at home

- Keep healthy foods more accessible

What To Expect While Switching?

Difficulties while changing to a new diet

When you start a new diet, you can feel a little nauseous at first. This is since your body may need some time to adjust to the new alterations. The incredible thing is that these negative effects are just temporary hurdles on your path to potential health, with most of them disappearing in 1-2 weeks.

Dietary changes may have the following side effects:

- Headaches
- Getting hungry
- Bloating or excessive gas
- Constipation
- Mood swings (irritability)
- Congestion or diarrhea

- Fatigue
- Dizziness
- Hunger pangs
- Concentration problems
- Disruptions in sleep
- Deficiencies in nutrition

These adverse effects are typically minor and only last a short time. However, if your symptoms continue, become severe, or include frequent vomiting, dizziness, or exhaustion, you should get medical help as soon as possible.

Why is it that switching our diet makes us feel uneasy?

The increased quantity of fiber and protein in the diet causes most of the adverse effects connected with altering the diet; however, occasionally, it's simply your brain needing caffeine or sweets.

Other factors that may cause irritation include:

- You're not getting enough calories.

- The diet is very restricted, with no fats, carbohydrates, or sweets allowed.

- You've cut out too many food categories from your diet.

- You are not getting enough nutrients from your diet.

- Your brain is yearning for the feel-good chemicals that your favorite meals provide.

- You're anticipating far too many beneficial improvements in your body, really too soon.

Common Mistakes to Avoid

1st Mistake: Trying to be perfect from the start

There is generally always one element that can be counted on. When individuals first begin following an alkaline diet, they strive for perfection. When they first start out, rationality vanishes as they strive to accomplish everything at once. This is undoubtedly true for most individuals when they begin making changes to their wellbeing or lifestyle, such as a diet program or gym routine. When you aim to be flawless from the start, you prepare yourselves for failure. When you're attempting to give up something, you have to deal with cravings, behavioral shifts, stress, psychological struggles, and trying to come up with alkaline foods to cook simultaneously.

Summary: Turning this weakness into a strength

- Don't attempt to accomplish everything at once, and don't aim to be great right away.

- Prioritize getting the Best in first, rather than limiting the BAD. This will render it more enjoyable and simple while still delivering tremendous results.

- When it comes to removing and switching away from harmful foods, take it one day & one week at a time: this week dairy, coming week caffeine. And don't go on to the next one since you've mastered the first.

- Focus on the Basics first: water, greens, oils, minerals, and moderate exercise are the 20% elements that will provide you 80% of the total benefit. When these five little modifications are added together, they add a significant advantage.

-

2ⁿᵈ Mistake: Lack of planning

Even the most veteran alkalizer will be undone by a lack of preparation. But, it's easy to be prepared. It's all about building a repertoire of simple, tasty alkaline meals that will become your go-to. Foods that you can rely on at any time.

Understanding what meals you'll eat in the coming days, planning ahead, and then, heaven forbid, buying the items you'll need to cook those meals are all part of being prepared. Everything is about a little forethought, planning, and preparation so that you may live alkaline comfortably and wonderfully.

Summary: Transforming this weakness into a strength

- Don't rely on the chance! If you live, shop, and eat daily, you will find yourself hungry, albeit with accessibility to acidic foods.

- A little planning makes a huge difference: plan your meals at least three days ahead of time and prepare for them!

- Always have a limited list of ingredients on hand — 8-10 items that you can prepare 5-6 easy alkaline snacks and meals at the stroke of a feather.

- Always have a few of 'get out of jail free' snacks on hand — nuts and seeds, sprout bread, avocados, and tomatoes are all good choices.

3rd Mistake: Digestion

The importance of the digestive system is underappreciated. Unfortunately, your digestive system becomes blocked and damaged after consuming an acidic, less-than-healthy diet for a long time. As a result, it becomes infected with yeast, germs, mycotoxins, and candida. Both of these scenarios are detrimental to your health and ambitions.

Worst of all, they'll imply that you're only reaping a small portion of the rewards of your efforts. So while being alkaline can help this cleaning process get started, there are several easy things you can really do to accelerate things - particularly if you're just getting started.

Summary: Converting this weakness into a strength

- Don't forget about your digestive system! Give it some love (particularly in the beginning), and the results will come in a flash!

- Green veggies, beans, chickpea, grapefruit, avocado, asparagus, and other high-fiber foods should be prioritized first.

- Simple carbohydrates, refined meals, processed foods, and other items that increase yeast growth in your digestive tract should be avoided.

- Get yourself some psyllium husks.

- Slow down, relax, and appreciate your food.

- Hydration, hydration, hydration.

4th Mistake: Quantities

This is a humorous yet truthful statement. The majority of individuals who begin an alkaline diet consume very little! For some reason, portions are thrown out the window, and they consume these tiny small meals. The greatest way to alkalize, cleanse, and heal the body and the digestive system is to saturate the body with nutrients, which you can only accomplish by eating a lot!

Summary: Turning it into an advantage

- Never miss a meal.

- Eat a lot

- If you're ever concerned, ensure you're getting adequate oils, complex carbohydrates, and proteins.

- Make 2x the lunch and dinner and store some for later use as snacks or a second serving if you become hungry after an hour or two.

- Appetite is acidic; therefore, don't allow it to happen to you.

- When you're initially starting out, have alkaline foods on hand at all times.

These four typical mistakes have all been working together to provide you with a compounding advantage. As a result, these four actions will provide you with a better reward than the finished product.

What To Expect Following the Dr. Sebi Lifestyle

Human bodies are generally acidic due to Western diets, which are high in fatty foods, excessive protein, not enough fiber, and too much sugar. Inflammation and a greater risk of numerous illnesses and disorders occur when the body gets overly acidic. On the other hand, an alkalizing diet helps balance your pH level, lowering acidity. Your body can thrive at its best when you live in more alkaline conditions. For example, alkalinity may help reduce inflammation in the brain, stomach, skin, and muscles, all of which are often affected in autistic children.

An alkalizing diet reduces inflammation and prevents the formation of yeast and harmful bacteria, which are frequent in autistic children. Detoxification is also improved as a result of this. When individuals follow the right alkalizing diet and detoxification procedure, many of them thrive. This is an example of a lifestyle modification that may make a huge difference in one's life. It's also crucial to figure out whether you have any dietary allergies or intolerance that might be causing your symptoms.

A healthy body comprises organs and functions that precisely control pH balance & sustain an alkaline condition. Rather than relying on fad diets and quick fixes, nutritionists recommend implementing long-term lifestyle modifications to achieve long-term success. This involves eating a nutrient-dense diet that contains foods from various food categories. In addition, limit your intake of highly processed foods, high in empty calories and low in nutritional content.

Tips for A Good Kickstart And a Longer Life

Eating a nutritious diet is something that most of us don't think about until we're in our mid-to-late-thirties. When we're young, we can usually "get away" with eating whatever we want whenever we want. As a result, some of us disregard the potential to develop good eating habits while still young. So don't be disheartened if you've had a poor day packed with too many yummy foods. Instead, make a note of what went wrong so you may learn from it.

1. Don't rely on your willpower to get things done. That's a lot of work. Instead, try to stay away from people, places, & programs to encourage you to consume unhealthy foods.

2. Increase your water intake. While we are hungry, we are frequently thirsty. So instead of grabbing for a candy bar, try sipping some water. Also, wherever feasible, drink water instead of sugary drinks.

3. Limit your selections. Limit the diet to select things to avoid consuming out of curiosity.

4. Include green veggies. Include a green or leafy vegetable in your meal.

5. Limit your intake of fatty dressings, sauces, and other condiments. Adding ranch dressing, crackers, cheese, and bacon to a salad become a fatty/high-calorie meal. Instead, eat a lot of veggies

6. Increase your intake of home-cooked meals. This is not only a healthy suggestion, but it is also cost-effective.

7. Order your food first if you're eating out. This will assist you in avoiding becoming influenced by the poor dietary choices of others.

8. Get plenty of rest. According to some studies, a Lack of sleep might boost your urge to eat. Because this is a difficult chore for some (due to family and/or professional responsibilities), take time to rest & unwind when you can. This might entail not watching television or using the Internet.

9. Discuss eating habits. & concerns with your doctor regularly during your consultations. Then, whenever it comes to health, there are no stupid questions.

10. Get started right away. Don't put off making New Year's Goals until January 1st. Immediate action has a lot of clouts.

Conclusion

Dr. Sebi's alkaline diet is credited for healing several disorders and maintaining the body in good condition. It's a low-fat, high-protein, high-fiber diet. It is high in alkaline foods, which aid in the healing of ailments and the body's overall wellness. Weight reduction, greater energy levels, improved brain function and clarity, and decreased cholesterol and blood pressure benefit from an alkaline food diet. Vegetable-based foods, such as veggies, grains, fruits, and certain legumes, make up a pH-balanced diet. Dr. Sebi's diet is based on restoring the body to its natural alkaline condition to maintain and improve health and fitness. It's an important part of his treatment strategy. It focuses on improving the body's capacity to rid itself of pollutants. It is possible to lower one's risk of becoming ill by adopting this diet. It uses common foods that have been shown to help treat conditions including cardiovascular disease, cancers, diabetes, and arthritis in health care goods.

As per Dr. Sebi, illness and disease are caused by mucus and can only thrive in an acidic environment. The alkaline diet is meant to make disease organisms uncomfortable and allow the body's immune system to heal and restore itself. Unfortunately, eating excessive meat and other animal-origin items and too many processed meals causes the body to become extremely acidic.

According to Dr. Sebi, we will be healthier if we eat a largely plant-based alkaline food diet. While eating meat, fish, or poultry on occasion would not kill you right away, it is also not beneficial long-term. Alkaline meals, such as those recommended by Dr. Sebi, are beneficial to body function and wellbeing since they restore the body's natural pH. The goal is to raise the pH of the blood to above 7.35 that will help you avoid degenerative illnesses and maintain your body working at its best. According to Dr. Sebi, our bodies need to be in alkaline conditions all of the time to be healthy and perform their functions successfully.

⭐ HAVE YOU LIKED IT? ⭐

To provide the best quality cases to customers, **I would love to hear your thoughts and opinions on my book.**

TO DO SO, I WOULD ENCOURAGE YOU TO <u>LEAVE A HONEST REVIEW ON AMAZON</u>.

The best way to do it? Uploading a brief video with you talking about the **#1** thing you liked the most about this book.

Is it too much for you? Not a problem at all! A simple written review is still an amazing thing!

<u>THANK YOU IN ADVANCE FOR YOUR VALUABLE FEEDBACK</u>. THIS WILL HELP ME A LOT AS A SELF-PUBLISHED AUTHOR.

Made in the USA
Las Vegas, NV
07 October 2023

78621088R00063